Clinical Practice of Emergency Medicine in US

美国急诊临床经验荟萃

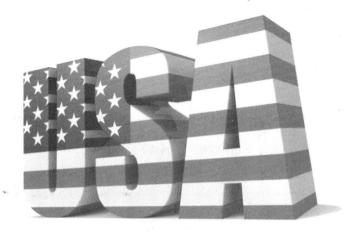

美国急诊
临床 365 问

(美)肖锋 / 编著

U0332155

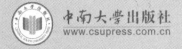
中南大学出版社
www.csupress.com.cn

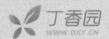
丁香园
WWW.DXY.CN

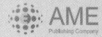
AME
Publishing Company

图书在版编目(CIP)数据

美国急诊临床365问/肖锋编著. —长沙:中南大学出版社,
2014.12

ISBN 978 - 7 - 5487 - 1238 - 1

Ⅰ.美... Ⅱ.肖... Ⅲ.急诊 - 美国 - 问题解答
Ⅳ.R4 - 44

中国版本图书馆 CIP 数据核字(2014)第 281433 号

美国急诊临床365问

[美]肖 锋 编著

□责任编辑	李 娴 孙娟娟	
□责任印制	易红卫	
□出版发行	中南大学出版社	
	社址:长沙市麓山南路	邮编:410083
	发行科电话:0731-88876770	传真:0731-88710482
□印 装	长沙市宏发印刷有限公司	

□开 本	720×1000 B5 □印张 13.5 □字数 262 千字	
□版 次	2015 年 1 月第 1 版 □2015 年 1 月第 1 次印刷	
□书 号	ISBN 978 - 7 - 5487 - 1238 - 1	
□定 价	48.00 元	

总　序

2008 年 4 月，美国急诊医师协会（American College of Emergency Physicians，ACEP）将急诊医学定义为：致力于诊断和治疗不可预见的疾病和外伤。2013 年 ACEP 对急诊医学临床模式（Model of the Clinical Practice of Emergency Medicine）进行了更新，进一步明确了急诊医学实践模式的三维内容，包括急诊医生的业务范畴（Physician Tasks）、患者病情判断（Patient Acuity），及急诊医学临床实践必须掌握的中心内容（Medical Knowledge，Patient Care，Procedural Skills）。国际急诊医学联盟（International Federation of Emergency Medicine，IFEM）认为急诊医学是一门临床学科，其知识和技能用以预防、诊断、治疗所有年龄的患者由于危重或急性疾病以及外伤导致的各类生理和行为紊乱；另外它还包括研究和发展院前及院内急诊医疗体系及其所需的技能。

总而言之，急诊医学兼具跨学科和综合性等专业特点。在任何一个国家和地区的医疗体系中，急诊科都是唯一一个处理所有有急性需求患者的前沿阵地。因此，作为一名急诊医生，一定要做到如下几点：知识要博而广；诊断要敏而全；治疗要精而准；操作要快而熟。

中国的急诊医学自 20 世纪 80 年代中期作为专科成立以来已经取得了突飞猛进的发展，但在专科建设、科室管理、人员（住院医师）培训、继续教育、临床实践等方面与美国相比还有很大的差距。与医学领域的其他学科相比，急诊医学尽管还很年轻，但其在循证医学方面的发展却日新月异。本系列丛书旨在通过 100 个真实的急诊病例（美国急诊临床病例解析 100 例）、200 个专题讨论（美国急诊临床必知 200 招）、365 个一日一题（美国急诊临床 365 问），向国内同仁及时介绍美国急诊临床标准化实践和基于循证医学的国际急诊医学的最新进展，对临床常见甚至罕见病例以及查房时最常遇到的问题提供科学的解答。同时，希望本系列丛书能够作为医学院临床实习生、各专科住院医生、基层医生、全科医生、危重病医生、急诊医生，以及任何到急诊科轮转或需要处理急诊病人的其他专科医生必备的参考书。

"美国急诊临床经验荟萃"丛书具备如下特色：

1. 循证：及时反映当前美国和基于循证医学的国际急诊医学新理念、新实践。

2. 短小：一题一答，一问一解，一个病例一个专题。

3. 易读：条理清晰、中英对照，是学习医学专业英语不可多得的辅助材料。

4. 实用：能够帮助临床医生解决实际的临床问题。

要了解和学习新的病例、新的必知和新的每日一题，可关注我的微信公共平台（美国急诊临床经验荟萃，或 Dr_XiaoUSA）、我的微博（微博名：Dr_XiaoUS），丁香园急救与危重病专栏（丁香园 ID：Dr_XiaoUS），以及我与《中华急诊医学杂志》和《中国急诊网》合作的专栏：马里兰大学医学院急诊科必知（http：//blog.sina.com.cn/s/articlelist_1904076233_14_1.html）。您也可以扫描下面的二维码直接关注。同时欢迎大家通过这几个平台或下面的电子邮箱进行反馈和交流。

感谢 Drs. Brian Browne，Laura Pimentel 和 Fermin Barrueto 对我的支持和帮助。感谢与我同舟共济 25 年的太太（徐燕）和我的两个可爱的儿子（Adam 和 Derek）对我的理解和支持。

Feng Xiao, MD
肖锋，医学博士
美国马里兰医学中心附属 Upper Chesapeake 医院急诊科
北京和睦家医院急诊科
fxiao88@gmail.com
2014 年 8 月 28 日于美国

前　言

　　《美国急诊临床365问》中的所有问题及答案均来自于美国最著名的、由临床急诊医生设计并为急诊医生服务的网络教育平台(EMedHome.com)中的"每日一题(Daily Question)"。每天，都有成千上万的来自世界各地的急诊医生访问这一平台。这一平台建立的目的，是通过提供既实用又具权威性的临床信息，以帮助急诊医生为病人提供更好和更安全的医疗服务。

　　本书选取的是 EMedHome.com 中 2013 年 4 月 22 日到 2014 年 4 月 24 日的"每日一题"的内容，并特地以中英对照的双语形式呈现给大家，是学习医学专业英语不可多得的辅助材料。为了能使大家能够更好地理解每一个问题，本人还对某些相关内容进行了展开讨论并配置了插图。

　　《美国急诊临床365问》的每一个问题都具有如下特点：①权威性和前沿性。使你能够在实践中应用最新的循证医学知识；②准确性。每一问都经过了急诊专家们的精心挑选和审查；③独立性。这些内容不受任何公司、药商或第三方的影响。

　　希望通过本书，可以帮助更多的人了解美国急诊相关的知识，掌握急诊相关的技能，更好地服务于患者，也更好地促进国内急诊医学的发展。

　　感谢 Dr. Rick Nunez 和 EMedHome.com 允许我将 Daily Question 的内容介绍给国内急诊医学的同仁以及广大读者。

Feng Xiao, MD

肖锋，医学博士

2014 年 8 月 28 日于美国

目录
CONTENTS

第四篇 **危重疾病篇**

第五篇 神经系统疾病篇

第六篇 **呼吸系统疾病篇**

第七篇 | 感染性疾病篇

第八篇 外科疾病与创伤篇

第九篇 | 肾脏疾病篇

第十篇 | 胃肠疾病篇

第十一篇 内分泌疾病篇

第十二篇 血液和肿瘤疾病篇

第十八篇 中毒性疾病篇

第十九篇 | 药物与治疗篇

第二十篇 | 环境与灾害性疾病篇

第二十一篇 | 其他疾病篇

1. 快速顺序插管

RSI, as originally conceived, is the simultaneous administration of sedative and paralytic with no ventilation-unless needed to prevent hypoxemia-while waiting for the paralytic to take effect. Why was RSI developed and applied to the ED?

按最初的设想，快速顺序插管(RSI)是指同时给予镇静和肌松药，在等待肌松药生效前没有必要进行人工通气，除非需要防止低氧血症。为什么会有 RSI 的产生及其在急诊科的应用?

RSI was developed by anesthesiologists for operative patients with high aspiration risk. This induction method has been adapted to the ED where all patients requiring airway management are assumed to be at aspiration risk.

RSI 是由麻醉医师为具有高误吸风险的手术患者所设计的，这一(麻醉)诱导方法已被急诊科采用，因为所有急诊科需要呼吸道管理的患者都必须被认为是高误吸危险人群(*Ann Emerg Med*, 2012, 59: 165)。

讨论: RSI 操作程序(6P)

Plan	确定方案
Position	患者头颈位置
Pre-Oxygenate	面罩供氧
Prepare	准备工作
Paralyze	给药后插管
Post-Intubation	插管后管理

2. 环状软骨加压的效果

Cricoid pressure is a routine component of rapid sequence induction and is designed to reduce the risk of reflux and its associated morbidity. Just how effective is application of cricoid pressure?

环状软骨加压是快速顺序插管的常规环节，旨在减少（食管）反流及其相关疾病的发病率。应用环状软骨加压效果如何？

A recent study of esophageal patency in volunteers utilizing MRI found that cricoid pressure by an experienced operator often resulted in lateral deviation of the esophagus and incomplete occlusion ofesophageal lumen.

最近一个在志愿者身上用磁共振观察食管开放程度的研究发现，由经验丰富的操作人员实施的环状软骨加压往往会使食管侧偏和食管管腔不完全闭塞，见图1所示（*J Emerg Med*，2012，42：606）。

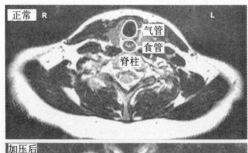
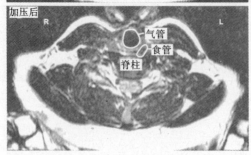

图1 环状软骨加压后（食管侧偏、管腔不完全闭塞）

3. 心肺复苏时气管插管后的通气频率

Following intubation during resusication of a cardiac arrest, how often should the provider deliver ventilations?

心脏骤停复苏过程中气管插管后,急救人员应该多久给一次通气?

Following placement of an advanced airway, the provider delivering ventilations should perform 1 breath every 6 – 8 seconds (8 to 10 breaths per minute) without pausing in applying chest compressions.

在气管插管后,管理呼吸道人员要在不影响胸外按压前提下,每6~8秒钟给一次通气(即每分钟8~10次)(*Circulation*, 2010, 122: S729)。

 ## 4. 心肺复苏时检查股动脉搏动

Clinicians frequently try to palpate arterial pulses during chest compressions to assess the effectiveness of compressions. Why must caution be exercised when relying on palpation of the femoral artery during CPR?

临床医生经常会在胸外按压时检查动脉搏动,以评估按压的有效性。为什么在心肺复苏(CPR)过程中检查股动脉时必须谨慎?

Because there are no valves in the IVC, retrograde blood flow into the venous system may produce femoral vein pulsations. Thus, palpation of a pulse in the femoral triangle may indicate venous rather than arterial blood flow.

由于下腔静脉没有瓣膜,股静脉血流逆行进入静脉系统可能会产生搏动。因此,在触诊股三角区时的搏动可能是静脉搏动而不是动脉搏动(*Circulation*, 2010, 122: S729)。

5. 美国院外心脏骤停的存活率

What is the survival rate of out-of-hospital cardiac arrest（OHCA）in the US? Given decades of research, how has the survival rate changed over the last 30 years?

美国院外心脏骤停(OHCA)的存活率是多少？经过几十年的研究，在过去30年里的存活率有什么改变？

OHCA has a survival rate of 9.6% in US; the survival rates after OHCA have remained virtually unchanged in the last 3 decades.

OHCA的存活率为9.6%，在过去的30年里，OHCA的存活率在美国实际上一直没有改变(*Critical Care*, 2013, 17：R235)。

 6. 美国院外心脏骤停在现场没有自主循环患者的存活率

Approximately 300, 000 persons experience cardiac arrest in the US annually. Survival to hospital discharge has increased to 9.6% with advances in care; however, if return of spontaneous circulation does not occur in the field, what portion survives?

美国每年约有30万人发生心脏骤停。随着急救技术的发展，出院存活率已提高到9.6%。但是，如果在现场自主循环(ROSC)没有恢复，那么存活率又是多少呢？

If return of spontaneous circulation does not occur in the field, only 0.9% individuals survive.

如果在现场自主循环(ROSC)没有恢复的话，只有0.9%的患者存活(*Ann Emerg Med*, 2014, 61：392)。

7. 美国院内心脏骤停出院存活率

Data from the National Registry of Cardiopulmonary Resuscitation database, the largest published database of in-hospital cardiac arrests, demonstrate what survival to discharge rate?

全国心肺复苏数据库(NRCPR)是美国最大的有关医院内心脏骤停的数据库，它的资料证明出院存活率是多少？

The registry demonstrated only an 18% survival to discharge rate.

全国心肺复苏数据库(NRCPR)的相关资料显示出院存活率只有18%（*Am J EM*, 2013, 31: 974）。

8. 除颤后是先进行心肺复苏还是先检查心律？

According to current ACLS guidelines, what is the immediate step following administration of a shock for VF/Pulseless VT?

根据目前最新的美国心脏协会心肺复苏指南(ACLS)，在对心室颤动或无脉搏室性心动过速的患者进行电击除颤后，紧接着的步骤应该是什么？

CPR should be resumed immediately after shock delivery (without a rhythm or pulse check and beginning with chest compressions) and continue for 2 minutes before the next rhythm check.

电击除颤后应立即恢复心肺复苏(不要检查心律或脉搏，直接开始胸外按压)，2分钟后再进行下一次心律检查（*Circulation*, 2010, 122: S729）。

9. 除颤时，放置除颤垫或除颤板的部位对除颤效果有影响吗？

Which position of placement of pads/paddles for defibrillation is most efficacious?

哪个部位放置除颤垫或除颤板是最有效的？

4 pad positions (anterolateral, anteroposterior, anterior-left infrascapular, and anterior-right-infrascapular) are equally effective to treat arrhythmias. Any of the 4 positions is reasonable for defibrillation.

4 个放置除颤垫的位置(前–外侧，前–后，前–左肩胛骨下和前–右肩胛骨下)有同样的治疗心律失常的效果。4 个位置中的任何一个都可用来电击除颤，见图 2(*Circulation*，2010，122：S706)。

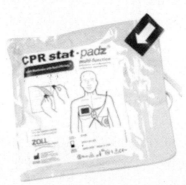

图 2　除颤垫

10. 孕妇心脏骤停剖宫产

Cardiac arrest in a pregnant patient with a fundal height at the level of the umbilicus (20 weeks) should prompt consideration of performance of a perimortem cesarean section. Is this procedure done only to try and save the baby?

如宫底高度在肚脐(孕 20 周)的孕妇发生心脏骤停,在行心肺复苏的同时,要及时考虑行剖宫产。这一操作仅仅是为了尽力挽救胎儿吗?

The mother may benefit as well. In one case series, 12 of 20 women had return of spontaneous circulation immediately after delivery.

行剖宫产是对胎儿的挽救,但对心脏骤停的孕妇也是有益的。在一组这种病例的系列报告中,20 个孕妇中有 12 个在剖宫产后立即出现自主循环恢复(*Emerg Med Clin N Am*, 2012, 30:949)。

11. 新生儿心肺复苏的胸外按压指征

What is the indication for the initiation of chest compressions when resuscitating a newborn?

对一个新生儿进行心肺复苏(CPR)时开始胸外按压的指征是什么?

Chest compressions are indicated for a heart rate that is < 60 per minute despite adequate ventilation with supplementary oxygen for 30 seconds.

胸外按压的指征为:在给氧和足够通气 30 秒钟后心率仍低于 60 次/min(*Circulation*, 2010, 122:S909)。

12. 新生儿脐带动脉搏动

Detecting the pulse of a newborn via palpation is most accurate at which site?

在检查新生儿动脉搏动时,什么部位最为准确?

The umbilical pulse.

脐带动脉搏动(*Circulation*, 2010, 122:S909)。

13. 新生儿心肺复苏通气频率

During resuscitation of a newborn, at what rate should assisted ventilations be delivered?

在新生儿心肺复苏的过程中，辅助通气的频率应该是多少？

40 to 60 breaths per minute.

每分钟 40 ~ 60 次（*Circulation*，2010，122：S909）。

14. 心肺复苏时碳酸氢钠的应用

The 2010 American Heart Association guidelines for ACLS do not recommend the routine use of sodium bicarbonate during CPR, except in 3 circumstances. Name them.

2010 年美国心脏协会心肺复苏指南中不建议常规使用碳酸氢钠，但下面 3 种情况除外，它们是哪 3 种情况？

The AHA guidelines for ACLS do not recommend the routine use of sodium bicarbonate during CPR, except for pre-existing metabolic acidosis, hyperkalemia, and tricyclic antidepressant intoxication.

除了已知患者存在代谢性酸中毒、高钾血症和三环类抗抑郁药中毒 3 种情况外，美国心脏协会心肺复苏指南（ACLS）不建议常规使用碳酸氢钠（*Am J EM*，2013，31：562）。

15. 能通过喉罩气道给药吗？

A laryngeal mask airway can be placed rapidly during CPR. In the absence of vascular access, can drugs be delivered via the LMA as they can via an endotracheal tube?

喉罩气道（LMA）能在心肺复苏中快速放置。在无血管通路的情况下，可以像通过气管内导管那样，通过 LMA 给药吗？

Delivery of drugs through the laryngeal mask airway to the pulmonary epithelium is unreliable and is not recommended.

通过喉罩气道（LMA）将药物送至肺上皮细胞是不可靠的，因此不建议使用喉罩气道（图3）给药（*N Engl J Med*，2013，369：e26）。

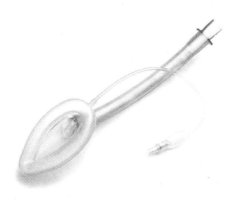

图3　喉罩气道

 # 16. 心脏震击猝死

The occurrence of commotio cordis depends upon the location of the blow to the chest. To induce VF, where must the blow occur?

心脏震击猝死综合征的发生取决于胸部受震击的位置，震击到什么位置才会诱发心室颤动（VF）？

To induce VF, the blow must occur directly over the center of the heart, not at the base, apex, or outside the precordium. The presence of a chest protector has not been correlated with decreased incidence or favorable outcome.

诱发心室颤动（VF），震击必须直接击至心脏的中心，而不是在心底、心尖或心前区之外，穿戴护胸与减少震击猝死综合征的发病率或好的预后没有关系（*J Emerg Med*，2014，46：e149）。

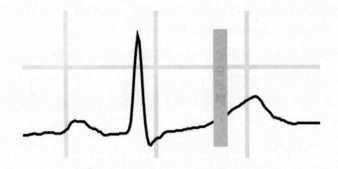

图4 心电图上 T 波峰值前的易颤期

讨论：

1. 心脏震击猝死综合征是无心脏疾病的年轻运动员发生胸前区撞击后出现心室颤动而导致猝死的原因之一。

2. 美国每年有 10～20 个新病例发生。

3. 心脏震击猝死的生存率在 20 世纪 70 年代为 10%，到 2012 年增加到 58%。

4. 在过去心脏震击猝死只与棒球运动有关，但现在也发生在冰球、垒球、曲棍球、空手道等对撞性激烈的运动项目中。

5. 心室颤动的发生与否取决于两个因素：
　①钝性震击的位置(见以上答案)。
　②钝性震击的时间：必须落在 T 波峰值前 10～40 毫秒之前的 20～30 毫秒瞬间之内(称易颤期)，这一窗口区大约占整个心脏周期的 6%(见图4)。

6. 抢救：根据 2010 年美国心脏协会心肺复苏指南(ACLS)制订的心室颤动方案。

 17. 高血镁造成的心脏骤停的治疗方法

What is the treatment of cardiac arrest and severe cardiotoxicity due to Hypermagnesemia?

由高血镁造成心脏骤停和严重的心肌毒性时的治疗方法是什么？

Administration of calcium (CaCL〔10%〕5 to 10 mL or calcium gluconate 〔10%〕15 to 30 mL IV over 2 to 5 minutes).

静脉注射 10% 氯化钙 5～10 mL 或 10% 葡萄糖酸钙 15～30 mL，2～5 分钟内

静脉注入（*Circulation*，2010，122：S829）。

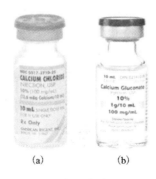

图 5   含钙类的制剂

（a）10% 氯化钙注射液；（b）10% 葡萄糖酸钙注射液

18. 低温造成心脏骤停的心肺复苏与血钾的关系

When resuscitating a patient in cardiac arrest from hypothermia, CPR should be considered to be futile if the serum potassium is above what level?

在对一个由低温造成的心脏骤停患者心肺复苏时，血钾高于什么水平可认为心肺复苏是徒劳的？

Termination of CPR should be considered when the serum potassium is above 12 mmol/L.

当血钾高于 12 mmol/L 时，应考虑终止心肺复苏（*N Engl J Med*，2012，367：1930）。

19. 你用超声指导心脏复苏吗?

Does the absence of cardiac activity on ultrasonography predict failed resuscitation in cardiac arrest?

可以用超声波显示没有心脏活动来预测心脏骤停复苏失败吗?

The current evidence does not support using ultrasonography alone to predict outcomes in cardiac arrest patients. A recent review yielded a survival to admission rate of 2.4% in patients with cardiac standstill. Of note, survival to admission is a poor surrogate for survival to discharge or neurologic outcomes.

目前证据还不支持只用超声波来判断心脏骤停患者的预后。根据一篇最新的文献综述,超声波下显示心脏停搏的患者的住院存活率为2.4%。值得注意的是,与出院存活率或神经恢复相比,住院存活率的临床意义要明显低很多(*Ann Emerg Med*, 2013, 62: 180)。

20. ST 段抬高型心肌梗死伴心源性休克或心衰与经皮冠状动脉介入治疗

In a patient with an acute STEMI and cardiogenic shock or acute severe HF, primary PCI may be performed up to how long following onset of MI?

对于一个急性 ST 段抬高型心肌梗死(STEMI, 图6)伴心源性休克或急性严重心衰的患者,紧急行冠状动脉介入(PCI)治疗,最长可以在心肌梗死后多久进行?

Primary PCI should be performed in patients with STEMI and cardiogenic shock or acute severe HF, irrespective of time delay from myocardial infarction onset.

不论心肌梗死发生的时间有多长,只要 ST 段抬高型心肌梗死(STEMI)患者伴有心源性休克或急性严重心衰都要进行紧急冠状动脉介入(PCI)治疗(*Circulation*, 2013, 127: 529)。

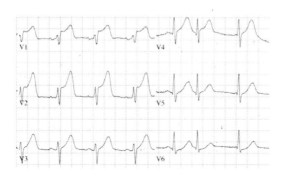

图6　ST 段抬高型心肌梗死心电图

21. 心肌梗死与超急性 T 波变化

Hyperacute T waves are early changes that may be seen on the EKG in an acute MI. How soon after coronary occlusion can hyperacute T waves appear?

超急性 T 波变化可以作为急性心肌梗死的早期心电图改变（图 7）。超急性 T 波可以在冠状动脉闭塞后多久出现？

Hyperacute T waves are noted as early as 30 min after the onset of coronary occlusion.

超急性 T 波可以在冠状动脉闭塞 30 分钟内出现（*J Emerg Med*, 2012, 43：e81）。

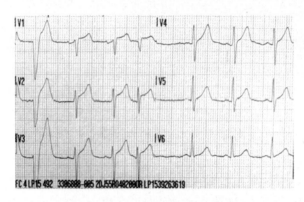

图 7　超急性 T 波变化心电图改变

？22. 非 ST 段抬高型心肌梗死与微栓塞

In non-ST-elevation acute coronary syndrome, the thrombus that occurs following plaque rupture is usually only partially occlusive. How, then, does ischemia and infarction occur?

对于非 ST 段抬高型急性冠状动脉综合征（ACS），斑块破裂形成的血栓通常只造成部分闭塞。那么，缺血和梗死是如何发生的？

In NSTE ACS, the thrombus is usually only partially occlusive but may cause intermittent downstream myocardial ischemia or downstream microvascular infarction due to microemboli.

非 ST 段抬高型 ACS 血栓通常只是部分闭塞，但可能会导致由微栓塞造成的间歇性区域内心肌缺血或微血管梗死（*J Emerg Med*, 2009, 36：162）。

23. 右室心肌梗死的特异性心电图改变

What EKG finding is pathognomonic for a right ventricular myocardial infarction?

什么样的心电图改变对右室心肌梗死(RVMI)具有特异性诊断意义?

Disproportionate ST segment elevation with greater ST elevation in lead III than in lead II is pathognomonic for an RVMI.

Ⅲ导联与Ⅱ导联 ST 段不对称地抬高,即Ⅲ导联 ST 段抬高比Ⅱ导联明显,是诊断右室心肌梗死(RVMI)的特异性改变,如图 8 所示(*Exp Clin Cardiol*, 2013, 18: 27)。

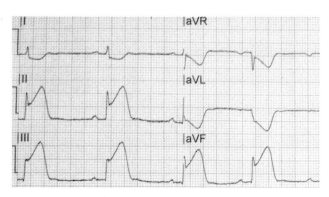

图8 右室心肌梗死的特异性心电图

24. 右室心肌梗死与 V4R

Which EKG lead demonstrates the greatest sensitivity and specificity for an RV infarct?

哪一个心电图导联在诊断右室心肌梗死时最敏感和最特异?

Right-sided precordial lead V4R demonstrates the greatest sensitivity and specificity for an RV infarct.

右侧胸前 V4R 导联对右室心肌梗死最敏感和最特异（*Mayo Clin Proc*，2010，85：e52）。

25. 镜像导联 ST 段压低在诊断 ST 段抬高型心肌梗死中的作用

By definition, reciprocal ST-depression should never occur in ECGs with narrow-complex STEMI mimics, with one notable exception. Name the exception.

根据定义，镜像导联 ST 段压低不应该发生在窄 QRS 波群、ST 段抬高型心肌梗死类似疾病的心电图上，但有一个例外，请指出这个例外是什么？

Reciprocal ST-depression should never occur in ECGs considered normal or those with narrow-complex STEMI mimics, except lead aVR with pericarditis.

镜像导联 ST 段压低应该永远不会出现在正常正电图或那些与 QRS 波群、ST 段抬高型心肌梗死(STEMI)类似疾病的心电图上，但在有心包炎时的 aVR 导联除外，如图 9 所示(*Am Heart J*，2010，160：995)。

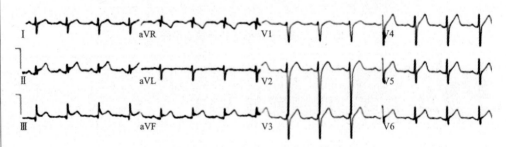

图9　心包炎时 aVR 导联显示的心电图

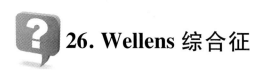 26. Wellens 综合征

Wellens' syndrome refers to ECG findings suggestive of significant LAD stenosis, and patients are at high risk for anterior wall MI. What are the findings? Must the patient have active chest pain to meet the criteria for Wellens' syndrome?

Wellens 综合征是指心电图提示有显著的左前降支狭窄，患者具有发生前壁心肌梗死的危险的情况。ECG 的变化是什么？患者必须有活动性胸痛才符合 Wellens 综合征的标准吗？

Wellens' syndrome = symmetric, deeply inverted or biphasic T waves in the anterior leads with preserved R wave progression, without pathologic Q waves and ST elevation. Pain is usually resolved at the time of these ECG changes.

Wellens 综合征的心电图变化是指胸前导联对称，深深倒置或双相 T 波，而 R 波还是渐进性增高，也没有病理性 Q 波和 ST 段抬高(图 10)。疼痛通常在出现这些心电图改变时缓解(*Am J Emerg Med*, 2013, 31: 439)。

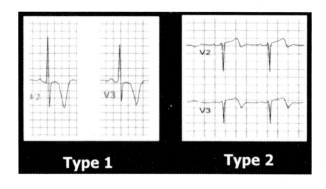

图 10　Wellens 综合征心电图

27. 不能口服阿司匹林时，如何应用阿司匹林？

Early administration of aspirin has been associated with decreased mortality in Acute Coronary Syndrome. How is aspirin ordered for patients with severe nausea, vomiting, or disorders of the upper GItract that make oral administration not feasible?

阿司匹林的早期应用一直与降低急性冠状动脉综合征的死亡率有关。对有严重恶心、呕吐或上消化道功能紊乱而不能口服的患者，如何应用阿司匹林？

Aspirin suppositories (300 mg) are safe and can be considered for patients with severe nausea, vomiting, or disorders of the upper gastrointestinal tract.

阿司匹林栓剂 300 mg(图 11)是安全的，可用于患有恶心、呕吐或上消化道疾病的患者(*Circulation*, 2010, 122: S787)。

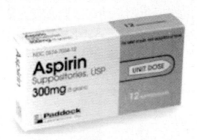

图 11　进口的阿司匹林栓剂

 ## 28. 为什么不能用硝酸甘油？

Name 4 contraindications to the use of nitrates in patients presenting with Acute Coronary Syndrome.

列出在处理急性冠状动脉综合征患者时禁忌使用硝酸甘油的 4 个指征。

According to AHA guidelines, hypotension (SBP < 90 mmHg or 30 mmHg below baseline), extreme bradycardia (<50 bpm), tachycardia without heart failure (>100 bpm) and presence of RV infarction are contraindications.

根据美国心脏协会（AHA）制订的指南，低血压（收缩压＜90 mmHg 或低于基线 30 mmHg），严重心动过缓（＜50 次／min），非心脏衰竭性心动过速（＞100 次／min）和右室心肌梗死是使用硝酸甘油的禁忌（*Circulation*，2010，122：S787）。

29. 服用达比加群酯患者出血的评估

What is the role of an APTT in assessing the degree of anticoagulation in a patient taking dabigatran who presents to the ED with bleeding?

在评估一个服用达比加群酯的患者因出血到急诊就诊时的抗凝程度时，活化部分凝血活酶时间（APTT）的作用是什么？

A normal APTT effectively rules out any significant dabigatran effect; however an elevated value gives little information as to the degree of anticoagulation.

正常的 APTT 可以有效地排除达比加群酯任何显著的致出血作用，但 APTT 值升高对抗凝程度的评估却没有什么意义（*EMedHome*，*Feature Article* 7/1/，2013）。

30. 心肌梗死再灌注后加速性室性自主心律

A patient is treated with IV thrombolysis for an acute MI. 90 minutes later he is clinically stable and pain free, but his EKG exhibits an accelerated idioventricular rhythm. What management is required?

一个急性心肌梗死的患者在静脉溶栓治疗 90 分钟后，临床稳定，无胸痛，但心电图呈现加速性室性自主心律（AIVR）。此时应如何处理？

AIVR is recognized as a "reperfusion dysrhythmia". Deterioration into a malignant ventricular dysrhythmia is rarely observed, and no specific treatment is required.

加速性室性自主心律（AIVR）被公认为是"再灌注后心律失常"（图 12）。它演变成恶性心室节律紊乱的情况并不多见，因此并不需要什么特殊的治疗（*J Emerg Med*，2011，41：182）。

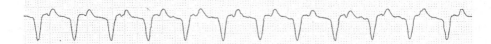

图 12　加速性室性自主心律心电图

 31. 紧急冠状动脉旁路移植术

Emergency coronary-artery bypass grafting (CABG) is required in what portion of coronary balloon angioplasty procedures?

紧急冠状动脉旁路移植术(CABG)在冠状动脉球囊血管成形术(PTCA)中所占的比例是多少?

Emergency CABG, which was initially required in 6% – 10% of procedures, has become a rare event, with an incidence of 0.1% – 0.4% in contemporary studies.

冠状动脉球囊血管成形术(PTCA)后需要紧急冠状动脉旁路移植术,这在过去约占 6% ~ 10%,现在已较为罕见,其需要率占 0.1% ~ 0.4%(*N Engl J Med*, 2013,368：1498)。

 32. 急性冠状动脉综合征患者的输血指标

According to current guidelines, transfusion should be considered for patients with active acute coronary syndromes with what hemoglobin level?

根据目前的指南,对有活动性急性冠状动脉综合征的患者进行输血的血红蛋白指标是多少?

Transfusion should be considered for inpatients with active acute coronary syndromes with an Hb level at or below 8 g/dL.

对有活动性急性冠状动脉综合征的患者进行输血的血红蛋白指标是等于或低于 8 g/L(*Hematology*, 2013,2013：638)。

33. 为什么中等大小的粥样硬化斑块更易破裂?

In many cases medium-size plaques (30% – 40% stenosis) are more likely to rupture than larger, more obstructive ones. This helps explain why stress tests and symptoms may not predict the risk of MI. Why are smaller plaques more vulnerable to rupture?

在很多情况下,中等大小(造成30% ~ 40% 血管管腔狭窄)的粥样硬化斑块要比大的和阻塞严重的斑块更容易破裂。这有助于解释为什么负荷试验和症状有时无法预测心肌梗死的危险。为什么小一点的斑块会更容易破裂呢?

Moderate plaques may be vulnerable because they are less mature, with a large lipid core and a thin cap prone to rupture, exposing the thrombogenic subendothelial components.

中等大小的粥样硬化斑块很脆弱,这是因为它们还没有成熟,大量的脂质核和薄的覆盖层很容易破裂,使血管内皮促血栓形成物得以暴露(*Clev Clin J Med*, 2014, 81: 233)。

 34. 冠状动脉夹层动脉瘤

If a young woman presents with apparent ACS (ST-segment elevation/depression, elevated troponin) without any risk factors, the clinician should have a high suspicion for what diagnosis?

如果一个年轻女性有明显的急性冠状动脉综合征指征(ST 段抬高或压低,肌钙蛋白升高)但无任何危险因素,临床医生应高度怀疑什么诊断?

Spontaneous coronary artery dissection, which occurs more commonly in women.

应高度怀疑自发性冠状动脉夹层动脉瘤,而且经常发生在女性 (*Am J Emerg Med*, 2013, 31: 1156. e1)。

讨论：

1. 自发性冠状动脉夹层动脉瘤多发生于年轻怀孕或服用避孕药的女性。

2. 可用血管内超声技术辅助诊断。

 ## 35. 心房颤动与心肌梗死

Is the presence of atrial fibrillation an independent risk factor for myocardial infarction?

心房颤动是诱发心肌梗死的独立危险因素吗?

A recent analysis of a large cohort of patients indicated that AF is independently associated with an increased risk of incident MI, especially in women and blacks.

最近的一项大型队列分析表明，心房颤动是增加心肌梗死的一个独立危险因素，尤其是在妇女和黑人中(*JAMA Intern Med*, 2014, 174: 107)。

 ## 36. 心力衰竭的克星：心脏再同步化治疗

What is the only heart-failure treatment that rapidly improves cardiac function and symptoms AND reduces long-term mortality?

什么是能够迅速改善心力衰竭患者心脏功能和症状，降低远期死亡率的唯一方法?

Cardiac-resynchronization therapy, in which biventricular stimulation reestablishes coordinated contraction in patients with ventricular dyssynchrony due to left bundle-branch block.

心脏再同步化治疗，也就是通过双心室刺激使由左束支传导阻滞导致的心室不同步重新建立起协调的收缩(*N Engl J Med*, 2014, 370: 1164)。

37. 窦性心动过速的上限

What is the upper limit of the rate of sinus tachycardia?

窦性心动过速的最高上限是什么？

The upper limit ofthe rate of sinus tachycardia is 200/min minus the patient's age.

窦性心动过速（图13）的最高上限是每分钟220次减去患者的年龄（*N Engl J Med*，2012，367：1438）。

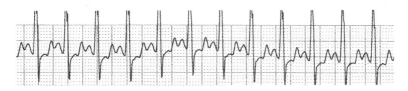

图13　窦性心动过速心电图

38. 咖啡因和心房颤动

Is it appropriate to caution a patient with a history of paroxysmal atrial fibrillation to avoid caffeine?

是否应该提醒阵发性心房颤动患者避免咖啡因？

There is a large body of scientific evidence to suggest that drinking moderate amounts of coffee and tea does not cause AF and may even decrease its occurrence.

有大量的科学证据表明，中等量饮用咖啡和茶，不会造成心房颤动，反而可能减少其发生（*Mayo Clin Proc*，2013，88：394）。

39. 心房颤动的转复与抗凝

For patients with atrial fibrillation of more than 48 hours' duration, therapeutic anticoagulation is recommended for how long before and after cardioversion?

心房颤动持续时间超过 48 小时的患者，心律转复前和转复后要有效抗凝治疗多长时间？

For patients with AF of >48 hours' duration, therapeutic anticoagulation for at least 3 weeks before and 4 weeks after cardioversion is recommended.

心房颤动持续时间超过 48 小时的患者，要在有效抗凝 3 周后才能进行心律转复，转复后还要继续抗凝 4 周(*Mayo Clin Proc*, 2013, 88:495)。

 40. 心房颤动自动转复的比例

What portion of patients with presumed recent – onset atrial fibrillation spontaneously convert to normal sinus rhythm within 2 – 3 days?

在新近发生心房颤动的患者中，有多少比例的患者会在 2 ~ 3 天内自动转复为正常窦性心律？

Approximately 2/3 of such patients spontaneously convert to NSR within 2 – 3 days.

大约会有三分之二的这样的患者会在 2 ~ 3 天内自动转复为正常窦性心律(*J Emerg Med*, 2012, 42:139)。

41. 多发性房性心动过速

Multifocal atrial tachycardia is characterized by a rhythm that is irregular; three abnormal P waves are necessary for the diagnosis. What is the pathophysiology of the etiology of MAT?

多发性房性心动过速(MAT)的特点是节律不规则(图 14);有 3 个异常的 P 波是重要的诊断条件。MAT 发生的病理生理学原因是什么?

MAT results from multiple atrial premature beats in an atrium poisoned by hypoxia, increased atrial pressure, and, theophylline. MAT is now uncommon because of the reduced use of theophylline.

MAT 是由于心房受缺氧、房内压增高和茶碱的影响而出现多源性房性期前收缩。由于茶碱应用的减少,MAT 已不多见(*N Engl J Med*, 2012, 367:1438)。

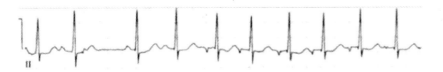

图 14　多发性房性心动过速心电图

讨论:

1. MAT 常见于哮喘、COPD、肺动脉高压和使用茶碱的患者。

2. 即使血压低也不要电击心律转复,应纠正低血容量、控制感染或治疗任何其他原因。

3. 可以静脉给硫酸镁。

42. 房性心动过速两个独特的特征

Emergency Physicians are commonly called upon to diagnose supraventricular tachycardias. What are two unique characteristics of atrial tachycardias?

急诊医师经常会遇到室上性心动过速。什么是房性心动过速的两个独特的特征?

Atrial tachycardias may occur in repetitive short bursts, and they are frequently characterized by a warm-up phenomenon in which the atrial rate increases slightly over the first 5 – 10 seconds before stabilizing.

房性心动过速可反复短时间出现,并常常在刚开始稳定前的5~10秒内心房频率略有增加,即所谓的"热身现象"(*N Engl J Med*, 2012, 367: 1443)。

43. 非持续性室性心动过速的最新定义

What is the current definition of nonsustained ventricular tachycardia?

非持续性室性心动过速(NSVT)的最新定义是什么?

The American College of Cardiology/AHA define NSVT as 3 or more wide QRS complexes, originating from the ventricles at a rate of more than 100 beats/min, that terminates spontaneously in less than 30 seconds.

美国心脏病学会/美国心脏协会将非持续性室性心动过速(NSVT)定义为3个或更多的起源于心室速度超过100次/min的宽QRS波群(图15),并且在30秒内自动终止(*Mayo Clin Proc*, 2012, 87: e87)。

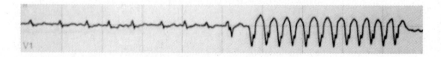

图15 非持续性室性心动过速

44. 不规则宽 QRS 心动过速

Stable wide-complex irregular tachycardias are almost always one of two arrhythmias. Name them.

稳定型不规则宽 QRS 心动过速几乎都是出现在两种心律失常之中（图 16）。它们是？

Atrial fibrillation with aberrancy or the Wolff-Parkinson-White syndrome.

心房颤动伴差异性传导或预激综合征（*N Engl J Med*，2012，367：1447）。

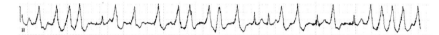

图 16　稳定型不规则 QRS 心动过速心电图

讨论：

1. 不规则宽 QRS 心动过速（心房颤动伴差异传导或预激综合征）的首选药物为普鲁卡因胺。

2. 不规则宽 QRS 心动过速不要用地高辛、β 受体阻滞药或钙通道阻滞药。

45. 儿茶酚胺多形性室性心动过速

What is catecholaminergic polymorphic ventricular tachycardia?

什么是儿茶酚胺多形性室性心动过速（CPVT）？

CPVT is an adrenergically mediated arrhythmia classically induced by exercise or emotional stress and found in structurally normal hearts. It is an important cause of cardiac syncope and sudden death in childhood.

CPVT 是一种肾上腺素能介导的心律失常(图17),通常是由运动或情绪紧张诱发,患者心脏结构正常。这是儿童发生心源性晕厥和猝死的一个重要原因(*Ped Emerg Care*,2011,27:1065)。

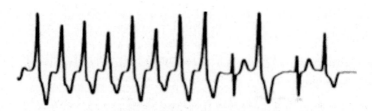

图 17　儿茶酚胺多形性室性心动过速心电图

讨论:

1. CPVT 是一种遗传性心律紊乱,发生率大概为 1:10000,平均发病年龄为 6~10 岁。

2. 临床表现:轻者可在情绪紧张或运动后出现心悸或头晕,重者可出现晕厥或猝死。

3. 诊断:家族史,典型表现,诱发试验(运动或儿茶酚胺试验),24 小时心电(Holter)监测。

4. 治疗:预防诱发因素,药物(β 受体阻滞药和钙通道阻滞药),植入型自动心脏除颤器(AICD)。如上述处理无效,可考虑行左侧颈交感神经切断术。

46. 单形性和多形性室性心动过速的意义

Why is the differentiation between monomorphic and polymorphic ventricular tachycardia important in terms of the underlying etiology of the arrhythmia?

为什么区分单形性和多形性室性心动过速对判断造成心律失常的病因非常重要?

Patients with monomorphic VT typically have structural heart disease, whereas patients with polymorphic VT characteristically have electrolyte abnormalities, a drug effect, ischemia, or a genetic cardiac channelopathy.

单形性室性心动过速患者通常有器质性心脏疾病,而典型的多形性室性心动过速患者可能是由电解质紊乱、药物作用、缺血或某种遗传性心脏离子通道病引起(*Mayo Clin Proc*,2008,83:1392)。

47. 校正后 QT 间期延长

What is considered a prolonged corrected QT interval on 12 – lead ECG?

在 12 导联心电图上，校正后 QT 间期延长是如何定义的？

The 99th percentile for QTc in adult males is 470 ms and in adult females 480 ms, with significant overlap between the normal spectrum and genetically affected individuals with no or only mild QT prolongation.

成年男性第 99 百分位的 QT 间期为 470 毫秒，女性为 480 毫秒，与正常和遗传上有轻度 QT 间期延长的人之间有显著重叠，见图 18（*Circulation*，2014，129：1524）。

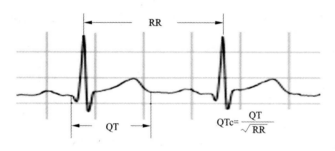

图 18　QT 间期与 QTc 的计算

 ## 48. 轻度至中度饮酒与心血管疾病

Observational studies consistently report that light to moderate drinkers are at lower risk for CV diseases than abstainers. What is the standard definition of light to moderate alcohol intake?

观察性研究报告一致认为轻至中度饮酒者与不嗜酒的人相比发生心血管疾病的风险较低。什么是轻度至中度的酒精摄入量？

第
三
篇

心
血
管
疾
病
篇

29

The standard definition of light to moderate alcohol intake is up to 1 drink/day for women and up to 2 drinks/day for men. Red wine, due to its array of nonalcoholic components, is associated with the best health outcomes.

轻度至中度的酒精摄入量的标准定义是女性每天 1 杯(14 g 乙醇量),男性每天最多 2 杯。红葡萄酒,由于其多种非乙醇性成分的作用,对健康是最有益处的(*Mayo Clin Proc*,2014,89:382)。

 49.嗜酒和室性心律失常

The association between alcohol and the occurrence of atrial fibrillation is well known ("holiday heart"). However, is there a relationship between alcohol intake and ventricular arrhythmias?

乙醇和发生心房颤动之间的关系是众所周知的(俗称"假日心脏")。然而,嗜酒和室性心律失常之间也有关系吗?

Excessive alcohol, whether from binge drinking or long-term heavy drinking, canstimulate ventricular arrhythmias. This effect of excessive consumption may be due to alcohol's tendency to cause QT interval prolongation.

过量饮酒,无论是酗酒还是长期大量饮酒,都可以诱发室性心律失常。过度嗜酒的危害可能是由于乙醇导致 QT 间期延长所致(*Mayo Clin Proc*,2014,89:382)。

 50.酒精与酒精性心肌病

Heavy alcohol consumption can result in alcoholic cardiomyopathy, which accounts for 1/3 of nonischemic dilated cardiomyopathy cases in the US. How much daily alcohol ingestion puts Individuals at risk for alcoholic cardiomyopathy and heart failure?

大量饮酒可导致酒精性心肌病,在美国占非缺血性扩张型心肌病的1/3。每天摄入多少乙醇量将会增加一个人酒精性心肌病和心脏衰竭的风险?

Individuals who consume more than 90 g of alcohol per day, which corresponds to about 7 drinks per day, for at least 5 years are at risk for the development of alcoholic cardiomyopathy and HF.

每天喝超过 90 g 乙醇的酒，大约相当于每天 7 杯，至少 5 年的人具有发生酒精性心肌病和心脏衰竭的危险(*Mayo Clin Proc*, 2014, 89: 382)。

 ## 51. 急性心内膜炎患者的血培养与抗生素

A febrile patient presents to the ED and you suspect acute endocarditis. Bearing in mind that Identifying the causative organism guides antimicrobial therapy, should you initiate empiric antibiotic therapy in the ED?

你怀疑一个急诊发热患者患有急性心内膜炎。一般来说，明确致病微生物可以指导抗生素治疗，那么，你应该在急诊科开始经验性抗生素治疗吗？

If patients are not acutely ill, avoid empiric antibiotic therapy until the organism is identified. If the patient is acutely ill, get 2 sets of blood cultures 30 – 60 minutes apart before starting antibiotics if possible.

如果患者病情不是很危重，在致病菌确定前可以不用抗生素治疗。如果患者危重，如可能，在 30~60 分钟的间隔内做 2 套血培养后可开始抗生素治疗(*Mayo Clin Proc*, 2013, 88: e145)。

 ## 52. 急性心内膜炎的首选抗生素

When initiating empiric antibiotic therapy in the ED for acute endocarditis, whatempiric antibiotics do you choose?

在急诊科对急性心内膜炎患者开始经验性抗生素治疗时，你会选择什么抗生素？

Give a 3rd or 4th-generation cephalosporin and an aminoglycoside (e. g. ceftriaxone & gentamicin) to cover likely organisms including MSSA and streptococci. If MRSA is suspected, monotherapy with vancomycin is initiated.

一种第三代或第四代头孢菌素加上一种氨基糖甙类的抗生素（如头孢曲松加庆大霉素），以覆盖可能的致病微生物，包括甲氧西林敏感金黄色葡萄球菌（MSSA）和链球菌。如果怀疑MRSA，可只用万古霉素（*Mayo Clin Proc*，2013，88：e145）。

 ## 53. 心内膜炎与脑磁共振成像

Even in the absence of neurologic symptoms patients with endocarditis may benefit from brain MRI. Why?

即使没有神经症状表现的心内膜炎患者也需要做脑部磁共振成像（MRI），为什么？

The majority of endocarditis patients have endocarditis-related cerebral lesions. These findings impact management (e. g. postponement of cardiac surgery in patients considered to be high risk for cerebral hemorrhage).

大多数心内膜炎患者伴有与心内膜炎相关的脑组织病变。这些病变的存在将影响治疗（例如对脑出血危险性高的患者要推迟心脏手术）（*J Emerg Med*，2012，43：e429）。

 ## 54. 感染性心内膜炎的关节损伤

Acute septic arthritis involving 2 or more joints should raise a suspicion of what condition?

累及2个以上关节的急性化脓性关节炎，应高度怀疑什么原因？

Acute septic arthritis involving 2 or more joints should raise a suspicion of Infective Endocarditis.

累及2个以上关节的急性化脓性关节炎，应高度怀疑感染性心内膜炎（*Mayo Clin Proc*，2007，82：615）。

55. 下腔静脉血栓形成导致腿部神经根症状和肌力减退

In a patient presenting with bilateral leg swelling with acute-onset low back pain with radiculopathy, the diagnosis of IVC thrombosis must be considered. What explains the radiculopathy and weakness in the legs that occurs with IVC thrombosis?

急性腰痛患者伴双下肢水肿和神经根刺激症状，必须考虑下腔静脉血栓形成。如何解释下腔静脉血栓形成导致腿部神经根症状和肌力减退？

The venous congestion in the venous plexus of the lumbar spine explains the radiculopathy and weakness in the legs, due to increased localized pressure around the L2 – L4 nerve roots.

腰椎静脉丛的静脉淤血使第 2 腰椎至第 4 腰椎(L2 ~ L4)神经根周围局部的压力增加，导致腿部神经根刺激症状和肌力下降(*J Emerg Med*, 2014, 46: 479)。

56. 深静脉血栓形成抗凝治疗后的效果

A patient has completed anticoagulant treatment for a proximal DVT of the lower extremity. Would you expect residual thrombosis to be visible on venous duplex ultrasound?

深静脉血栓形成的患者已完成了抗凝治疗。你认为静脉多普勒超声检查还会看到残余的血栓吗？

More than half of patients with proximal DVT have residual vein thrombosis on VDUS 6 months – 1 year after completion of therapy. In fact, the presence of residual DVT has been shown to be a risk factor for recurrent VTE.

一半以上的深静脉血栓形成(DVT)患者在完成治疗 6 个月到 1 年后，在其静脉多普勒超声检查上还可见残留的静脉血栓。事实上，残余 DVT 的存在已经被证明是静脉血栓栓塞复发的危险因素(*Circulation*, 2014, 129: 917)。

57. 深静脉导管与血栓形成

Are peripherally-inserted central catheters or centrally-inserted catheters associated with a greater risk for deep vein thrombosis?

经外周置入中心静脉导管（PICC）和中心静脉导管（CVS），哪一个造成深静脉血栓形成的风险更大？

PICC are associated with a higher DVT risk than CVCs, especially in critically ill patients or those with a malignancy. In a recent meta-analysis, PICC were associated with an increased risk of DVT with an OR of 2.55 but not PE.

PICC 与 CVS 相比有更高的造成深静脉血栓形成的风险，尤其是那些危重症或有恶性肿瘤的患者。在最近的一项荟萃分析中，PICC 可增加深静脉血栓[（不是肺栓塞（PE）]形成的风险，其比值比为 2.55（*Lancet*，2013，382：311）。

58. 由导管引起的肢体深静脉血栓形成如何处理？

You diagnose an acute upper extremity DVT on a patient presenting to the ED who has a central venous catheter in place. Is anticoagulation required? Should you remove the catheter?

你发现一个留置有中心静脉导管的患者发生（同侧）急性上肢深静脉血栓形成（DVT）。是否需要抗凝？应该将导管拔除吗？

For patients with a catheter-related upper extremity DVT, anticoagulation is indicated, typically for 3 months. Catheter retrieval is not necessary as long as it remains functional and required for clinical care.

对于由导管引起的上肢 DVT，通常要进行为期 3 个月的抗凝治疗。只要导管功能正常，临床上又有留置的必要，可以不拔除（*Mayo Clin Proc*，2014，89：394）。

59. 股浅静脉血栓形成需要抗凝治疗吗?

You are evaluating a patient for a possible DVT of the leg and order a venous ultrasound. The radiology report notes that there is thrombosis in the superficial femoral vein. Does this require anticoagulation?

你在看一个可能有下肢深静脉血栓形成(DVT)的患者,并做了静脉多普勒超声检查,超声科报告有股浅静脉血栓形成。这个患者需要抗凝治疗吗?

The superficial femoral vein is actually a deep vein that is the continuation of the popliteal vein; it joins the profunda femoral vein to form the common femoral vein. Thrombosis warrants treatment as for any DVT.

股浅静脉实际上是一条深静脉,即腘静脉的延续,回流到股深静脉形成股总静脉。对股浅静脉血栓应该进行与任何其他深静脉血栓形成一样的治疗(*Circulation*, 2014, 129: 917)。

60. 炎症性肠病和静脉血栓栓塞

What is the relationship between inflammatory bowel disease and risk of venous thromboembolism?

炎症性肠病和静脉血栓栓塞形成之间有什么关系?

Multiple large studies have demonstrated that CD (and also ulcerative colitis) patients have a 1.5 - 3.5 - fold higher risk of incurring VTEs when compared with non-IBD patients.

多个大规模研究已经表明,与非感染性肠病相比,克罗恩病和溃疡性结肠炎的患者发生静脉血栓的风险要高 1.5 ~ 3.5 倍(*J Acute Med*, 2013, 3: 132)。

61. 手术或外伤后静脉血栓栓塞的治疗

You diagnose an ED patient with a first occurrence of a venous thromboembolism that occurs in the context of a transient risk factor (e. g. surgery or trauma). The patient asks for how long he has to be anticoagulated. What is the correct answer?

你发现一个急诊科患者在一次短暂的危险因素(例如手术或外伤)后出现了第一次静脉血栓栓塞。患者问他必须接受抗凝治疗多久。正确的回答应该是什么?

A first VTE that occurs in the context of a transient risk factor (such as surgery or trauma) has a very low risk of recurrence and 3 months duration is adequate.

在一次短暂的危险因素(例如手术或外伤)后出现的第一次静脉血栓栓塞复发的可能性很低,3个月时间的抗凝治疗就足够了(*Hematology*, 2013, 2013: 457)。

62. D – 二聚体诊断静脉血栓栓塞

What is the current estimated sensitivity and specificity of D-dimer assays validated in VTE patients?

D – 二聚体目前在诊断静脉血栓栓塞(VTE)患者时的可预计敏感性和特异性是多少?

D – dimer assays validated in VTE patients generally have sensitivities in the mid –90% range and specificities in the mid –40% range. Given these properties, the value of the D-dimer resides with a negative test.

在 VTE 患者中 D – 二聚体测定的敏感性通常在 95% 左右,特异性在 45% 左右。鉴于这些特性,D – 二聚体的价值在于阴性结果。如结果为阴性,可排除 VTE(*Hematology*, 2013, 2013: 457)。

63. 造成下肢静脉血栓的髂静脉压迫综合征

Among acute DVT patients who might be expected to realize substantial benefit from thrombolysis are those with occluded veins as a result of May-Thurner syndrome. What is the cause of this syndrome?

对溶栓疗法可能会相当有效的急性深静脉血栓形成患者中包括那些由髂静脉压迫(May-Thurner)综合征引起的静脉阻塞患者。髂静脉压迫综合征的病因是什么?

May-Thurner, or iliac vein compression, syndrome results from left common iliac vein compression by the right common iliac artery, which increases the risk of DVT in the left leg.

髂静脉压迫(May-Thurner)综合征是由于右髂总动脉对左髂总静脉的压迫所造成的,此综合征可增加左下肢深部静脉血栓形成的风险(*J Emerg Med*, 2013, 45: 244)。

64. 如何开始深静脉血栓形成的抗凝治疗?

In patients diagnosed with acute DVT of the leg, early initiation of Vitamin K antagonist therapy is recommended along with parenteral anticoagulation. For how long is parenteral anticoagulation continued?

患者在确诊为下肢急性深部静脉血栓形成后,维生素 K 拮抗药(华法林)治疗要早期与肠外(静脉或皮下肝素或低分子肝素)抗凝同时开始。肠外抗凝要持续多久?

Parenteral anticoagulation is continued for a minimum of 5 days and until the INR is 2.0 or above for at least 24 hrs.

肠外抗凝至少要持续 5 天,直到国际标准化比率(INR)达到 2.0 或以上并超过 24 小时(*CHEST*, 2012, 141(2_suppl): e24S)。

65. 轻度华法林过量

With non-life-threatening bleeding, a supratherapeutic INR of < 5 may be controlled by a temporary discontinuation of warfarin. If a patient has an INR of 2 – 3 (therapeutic range for nonvalvular AF), how long will a return to normal coagulation take?

在国际标准化比率(INR)小于 5 的情况下,出现的不危及生命的出血可以通过暂时停用华法林来控制。如果患者的 INR 为 2~3(非瓣膜性心房颤动的治疗标准),停药后多久会恢复到正常凝血状态?

Warfarin has a half-life of 1.5 to 2 days, so that if a patient has an INR of 2 to 3 a return to normal coagulation will take 4 to 5 days after discontinuation.

华法林的半衰期为 1.5~2 天,因此,如果患者的国际标准化比率(INR)为 2~3,停药后通常需要 4~5 天的恢复才能达到正常的凝血状态(*J Emerg Med*,2013,45:467)。

 66. 低分子肝素与华法林

You diagnose a patient with a proximal LE DVT. The DVT has occurred in the setting of known metastatic lung CA. Do you arrange for initiation of warfarin with LMWH until the INR is therapeutic?

你发现一个转移性肺癌患者发生下肢近端深部静脉血栓。你会计划开始给予华法林与低分子肝素治疗直到国际标准化比率(INR)达到治疗水平吗?

LMWH is preferred for the first 6 months as monotherapy in patients with proximal DVT/PE in patients with advanced or metastatic cancer.

6 个月单独应用低分子肝素在治疗晚期或转移性癌伴近端深部静脉血栓或肺栓塞(DVT/PE)时是首选的治疗方法(*Nat Comp Cancer Guidelines*,*Cancer-associated VTE.*,2013)。

67. 颈内动脉夹层的典型临床表现

Unilateral headache, focal cerebral ischemic symptoms, and partial Horner syndrome is the classic presentation of what entity?

单侧头痛、局灶性脑缺血症状、部分 Horner 综合征是什么疾病的典型表现？

Internal carotid artery dissection.

颈内动脉夹层（*J Emerg Med*，2011，41：43）。

68. 椎动脉夹层与颈痛

Vertebral artery dissection is a significant cause of stroke in young persons; up to half develop anterolateral neck pain as the initial complaint. What is the median time from onset of neck pain to the occurrence of posterior circulation symptoms?

椎动脉夹层是年轻人脑卒中的一个重要原因；约一半的患者会以颈前侧部位疼痛为首发症状。从颈部疼痛到后支循环症状出现的中位数时间是多久？

The median interval between the onset of neck pain and the occurrence of posterior circulation symptoms is typically 2 weeks.

从颈部疼痛到后支循环症状出现的中位数时间通常为 2 周（*J Emerg Med*，2011，40：151）。

69. 疼痛性 Horner 综合征

Horner syndrome comprises miosis, ptosis (Muller muscle paralysis), and anhidrosis ipsilateral to a lesion along the oculosympathetic pathway. What is the most common cause of a painful Horner syndrome?

Horner 综合征包括眼交感神经通路病变同侧出现瞳孔缩小，眼睑下垂（穆勒肌麻痹），无汗。一个伴有疼痛的 Horner 综合征最常见的原因是什么？

An internal carotid artery dissection is the most common cause of a painful Horner syndrome. This can present with an ipsilateral headache, commonly at the temple, eye, or throat.

颈内动脉夹层（动脉瘤）是伴有疼痛的 Horner 综合征最常见的一个原因。它同时表现为同侧头痛，通常在颞部、眼睛或咽喉（*J Emerg Med*, 2013, 45：252）。

 70. 急性腹主动脉闭塞的原因

Acute occlusion of the abdominal aorta is a potentially catastrophic vascular emergency with mortality as high as 75% in some series. What are the causesof acute occulsion of the abdominal aorta?

急性腹主动脉闭塞是一个潜在的灾难性的血管系统急症，有文章报道死亡率高达 75%。急性腹主动脉闭塞的原因是什么？

Acute occlusion can be the result of in situ thrombosis, saddle embolism, thrombosis of an abdominal aortic aneurysm, aortic dissection, or traumatic aortic hematoma (JEM, Vol. 44, 161).

导致急性腹主动脉闭塞的原因可能有原位血栓形成，马鞍状栓塞，栓塞性腹主动脉瘤，主动脉夹层，或创伤性主动脉血肿（*J Emerg Med*, 2013, 44：161）。

 71. 脾动脉瘤破裂

Although rare, splenic artery aneurysm ruptures are an important cause of hemoperitoneum and hypovolemic shock. Over 95% of cases occur in what patients?

脾动脉瘤破裂虽然罕见，但脾动脉瘤破裂是腹腔积血和引起低血容量性休克的一个重要原因。超过 95% 的病例发生于哪些患者？

Most splenic artery aneurysm are asymptomatic. Rupture occurs in 2% – 3% of cases, and 95% of these are in young pregnant women.

大多数脾动脉瘤是无症状的。只有 2% ~ 3% 的患者会出现破裂，其中 95% 发生于年轻的怀孕妇女（*J Emerg Med*, 2014, 46: e65）。

 ## 72. 未破裂的腹主动脉瘤的修复指征

What are the indications for repair of an unruptured abdominal aortic aneurysm (AAA)?

未破裂的腹主动脉瘤（AAA）修复的适应证有哪些？

Rapidly growing aneurysms (e. g. the AAA enlarged by >0. 7 cm in 6 months or 1. 0 cm in 1 year), those that reach 5. 5 cm in diameter, and those that become symptomatic should be repaired.

对快速增长的，如腹主动脉瘤（AAA）在 6 个月增大超过 0. 7 cm，或在 1 年内超过 1. 0 cm，直径达到 5. 5 cm 和那些有症状的 AAA 应进行修复（*Mayo Clin Proc*, 2013, 88: 905）。

 ## 73. 主动脉夹层动脉瘤会无痛吗？

Acute chest pain is the most common initial presentation of aortic dissection. Does painless acute AD commonly occur?

急性胸痛是主动脉夹层动脉瘤最常见的初发表现。会有无痛性的急性主动脉夹层动脉瘤发生吗？

Although acute chest pain is the most common initial presentation of AD, up to 17% of patients present without pain.

虽然急性胸痛是主动脉夹层动脉瘤最常见的起始表现，但高达 17% 的患者可能就诊时并无疼痛（*Am J Emerg Med*, 2013, 31: 1279）。

74. 真菌性动脉瘤

What is a mycotic aneurysm? What is the most common location?

什么是真菌性动脉瘤？最常见的部位在哪里？

A mycotic aneurysm is an aneurysm that results from an infectious process that involves the arterial wall. The aorta is the most common site of mycotic aneurysm, followed by the femoral, cerebral, and visceral arteries.

真菌性动脉瘤是一种动脉壁慢性感染过程所致的良性肿瘤。主动脉真菌性动脉瘤是最常见的部位，其次是股动脉，脑和内脏动脉（*J Emerg Med*, 2013, 45: e133）。

讨论：

真菌性动脉瘤的治疗主要包括应用抗生素和手术摘除。

75. 动脉导管未闭

Patent ductus arteriosus occurs in 1 in 2000 full-term infants. The ductus typically closes within 24 – 48 h of neonatal life. Rarely, an untreated PDA persists to adulthood resulting in CHF. A PDA is a vascular connection between what 2 structures?

动脉导管未闭（PDA）在 2000 个足月新生儿中会出现 1 个。胎儿出生后动脉导管通常在出生后 24 ~ 48 小时内关闭。在极少数情况下，未经治疗的 PDA 持续到成年而导致心力衰竭。PDA 是连接哪两个结构的血管？

Patent ductus arteriosus is a congenital cardiac condition in which the vascularconnection between the descending aorta and the pulmonary artery fails to close after birth.

动脉导管未闭是指连接降主动脉与肺动脉之间的血管在出生后仍没有关闭的一种先天性心脏病（*J Emerg Med*, 2013, 45: e193）。

76. 如何防止呼吸机相关性肺炎

Ventilator-associated pneumonia carries significant morbidity and variable mortality. At least half of all cases of VAP are considered preventable. Name 3 interventions readily implemented in the ED that can reduce rates of VAP.

呼吸机相关性肺炎(VAP)有很高的发病率和不同程度的死亡率。至少有一半的 VAP 病例被认为是可以预防的。指出 3 个在急诊科很容易采取的能够减少VAP 发生率的方法。

Interventions that may result in reductions in VAP rates include routine suctioning above the endotracheal cuff, elevating the head of the bed at least 30 degrees, and providing oral hygiene with 1.5% hydrogen peroxide.

可能减少 VAP 发生率的措施包括常规吸取气管导管气囊以上的分泌物,将床头抬高至少30 度,和用1.5%的过氧化氢溶液清洁口腔(*Ann Emerg Med*, 2014,64:299)。

讨论:肺炎的分类

社区相关肺炎(CAP)	不属于任何其他类型的肺炎
医疗相关性肺炎(HCAP)	90 天内在急性病医院住院超过 2 天 住在养老院或长期护理院 30 天内用过抗生素,进行过化疗或伤口护理 血液透析 家庭药物注射或伤口护理 家庭成员有多药抵抗菌感染 免疫力极度低下
医院相关肺炎(HAP)	住院两天后
呼吸机相关肺炎(VAP)	气管插管或气管切开两天后

77. 糖尿病酮症酸中毒与前列腺素

What is the cause of the nausea, vomiting, and abdominal pain that are seen frequently at presentation of diabetic ketoacidosis, especially in children?

恶心、呕吐、腹痛是糖尿病酮症酸中毒(DKA)常见的临床表现，尤其在儿童患者中。造成这些症状的原因是什么？

The increase in circulating prostaglandins-one of the metabolic derangements associated with DKA-is felt to be the cause of the nausea, vomiting, and abdominal pain.

血液中前列腺素水平的增加———一个与 DKA 相关的代谢紊乱因子，被认为是造成恶心、呕吐、腹痛的原因 (*J Emerg Med*, 2010, 39：449)。

 78. 糖尿病酮症酸中毒的严重合并症：脑水肿

Cerebral edema is a potentially devastating consequence of DKA. Risk factors for cerebral edema include younger age (especially < 5 years old). When does cerebral edema typically present after initiation of therapy?

脑水肿是糖尿病酮症酸中毒(DKA)潜在的死亡率极高的合并症。脑水肿的危险因素包括年龄小(特别是 5 岁以内)。脑水肿通常在治疗开始后什么时间内出现？

Cerebral edema typically presents 4 – 12 h after initiation of therapy. Early signs include headache, recurrent vomiting and confusion. Sustained unexpected lowering of heart rate should raise suspicion for cerebral edema.

糖尿病酮症酸中毒(DKA)合并的脑水肿通常在开始治疗后 4 ~ 12 小时出现。早期迹象包括头痛、频繁呕吐和神志恍惚。意想不到的持续性心率降低，应高度怀疑合并有脑水肿(*J Emerg Med*, 2013, 45：797)。

讨论：

死亡率	DKA 儿童伴脑水肿的死亡率是 20% ~ 30%
	在幸存者中，15% ~ 35% 会出现永久性神经系统障碍
治疗	减少液体输入量
	20% 甘露醇 0.25 ~ 1 g/kg，20 分钟内静脉注射
	3% 氯化钠注射液 5 ~ 10 mL/kg，30 分钟内静脉注射
	呼吸支持

 79. 为什么治疗过敏性休克时静脉滴注肾上腺素要慢速？

When administering an IV epinephrine infusion in the ED, such as for a patient with anaphylaxis, why is a slow infusion rate associated with fewer adverse effects?

在急诊科给予静脉滴注肾上腺素治疗过敏性休克的患者时，为什么慢速输液会减少不良反应的产生？

Slow infusion rates mainly affect Beta-receptors, whereas rapid infusion leads toalpha-receptor effects. Thus, a low dose and slow infusion produces bronchodilation and moderate BP increases without as many adverse effects.

缓慢滴注速度主要影响 β 受体，而快速输液会产生 α 受体的作用。因此，低剂量和静脉缓慢滴注在产生支气管扩张和中度的血压增高情况下，没有太多的不良反应(*Am J Med*，2014，127：S34)。

 80. 多巴胺可造成免疫抑制

In most cases, when a vasopressor is selected for the treatment of shock, norepinephrine-not dopamine-is considered the vasopressor of first choice. It is now believed that dopaminergic stimulation has undesired endocrine effects. What are they?

在大多数情况下，当决定治疗休克需要用升压药时，应用去甲肾上腺素而不是多巴胺。去甲肾上腺素被认为是首选的血管加压药。现在认为多巴胺系统的刺激可以产生不良的内分泌作用。为什么？

Dopaminergic stimulation may have undesired endocrine effects on the hypothalamic-pituitary system, resulting in immunosuppression, primarily through a reduction in the release of prolactin.

多巴胺系统兴奋可能会对下丘脑－垂体系统有不良的内分泌影响，主要是通过减少泌乳素的释放造成免疫抑制（*N Engl J Med*, 2013, 369: 1726）。

 81. B 型乳酸性酸中毒

What is a type B lactic acidosis?

什么是 B 型乳酸性酸中毒？

Type B lactic acidosis is characterized by elevated lactate without evidence of tissue hypoperfusion. metformin-associated lactic acidosis would be one example.

B 型乳酸性酸中毒的特点是没有组织低灌注前提下的乳酸水平升高。长期服用二甲双胍造成相关的乳酸性酸中毒，就是一个例子（*J Emerg Med*, 2011, 40: 271）。

讨论：乳酸血症分类

类型	A 型	B 型
定义	组织灌注不足或低血氧症	无组织灌注不足或低血氧症
原因	产生过多的乳酸 消耗减低	B1：肝病，肾病，糖尿病，肿瘤 B2：药物或毒素 B3：遗传病

 82. 血清乳酸水平升高与死亡率的关系

What is the significance of an elevated serum lactate level in a patient presenting to the ED with a clinically suspected infection with a normal blood pressure?

一个血压正常但临床疑似感染的急诊科患者血清乳酸水平升高的意义是什么？

Recent studies indicate that elevated lactate levels are associated with mortality independent of shock.

最近的研究表明，无论患者有无休克，乳酸水平升高与死亡率相关，见图 19

(*Mayo Clin Proc*, 2013, 88: 1127)。

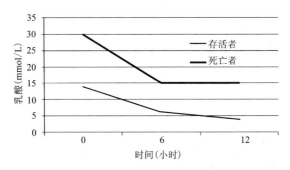

图 19　血清乳酸水平与死亡率的关系

 83. 严重脓毒症与乳酸清除率

How is lactate clearance used to assess initial response to resuscitaiton in severe sepsis?

如何用乳酸清除率来评估严重脓毒症对复苏的初步反应？

The best available evidence suggests that lactate clearance of at least 10% at a minimum of 2 hours after resuscitation initiation is a valid way to assess initial response to resuscitation in severe sepsis.

目前有证据表明，复苏开始后 2 小时内至少 10% 的乳酸被清除（图 20），是一个有效的评估严重脓毒症对复苏有初步反应的方法（*Acad Emerg Med*, 2013, 20: 844）。

讨论：血清乳酸清除率与死亡率的关系

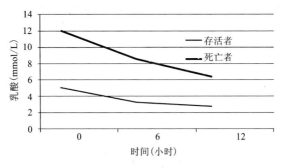

图 20　血清乳酸清除率与死亡率的关系

84. 脓毒症最初液体复苏量

Because most patients presenting with sepsis are volume depletion, an empiric fluid bolus for any patient with suspected severe sepsis with hypotension or an elevated lactate level >4 mmol/L is recommended. How much of a bolus should be given?

由于大多数脓毒症患者都是血容量不足，因此，对任何怀疑严重脓毒症患者伴低血压或血清乳酸水平升高 >4 mmol/L 都应给予液体快速输注。应给多大量的液体？

According to the 2012 Surviving Sepsis guidelines, an initial 30 mL/kg crystalloid bolus is administered.

根据 2012 年"战胜脓毒症"指南，最初要快速给予 30 mL/kg 的晶体液（*Ann Emerg Med*, 2014, 63：35）。

讨论：严重脓毒症或脓毒性休克 3 小时内复苏措施（复苏模块）

静脉晶体液（30 mL/kg）

在给予抗生素前抽血培养

静脉滴注广谱抗生素（对严重脓毒症或脓毒症感染性休克者要在 1 小时之内应用）

测量血清乳酸水平

 85. 去甲肾上腺素在脓毒性休克中的作用

Norepinephrine is now considered the vasopressor of choice for most cases of septic shock. What are the effects of NE on mean arterial pressure, stroke volume, and cardiac filling pressures?

去甲肾上腺素（NE）现在被认为是治疗大多数感染性休克的首选升压药。NE 对平均动脉压（MAP），心每搏排血量和心脏充盈压有什么影响？

NE is a potent alpha-adrenergic agonist with less Beta-agonist effect; it increases MAP by vasoconstriction, with a small (10 – 15%) increase in CO and stroke volume. Filling pressures are unchanged or modestly increased.

去甲肾上腺素(NE)是一个强有力的 α 肾上腺素受体激动药和较小的 β 受体激动剂;它通过血管收缩作用增加 MAP,同时也可使心排血量和每搏排血量增加 10% ~ 15%。心脏充盈压将保持不变或有小幅度增加(*Am J Respir Crit Care*, 2011, 183: 847)。

 86. 休克时去甲肾上腺素可降低死亡率

Current research suggests that norepinephrine confers mortality benefit as compared to dopamine in which subgroup populations in shock?

目前研究表明,应用去甲肾上腺素对哪种休克患者要比多巴胺有较好的降低死亡率的作用?

There is no significant difference in mortality between NE and dopamine in heterogeneous populations of hypotensive shock. Current research suggests that NE confers mortality benefit in cardiogenic and septic shock.

对所有低血压休克患者来说,应用去甲肾上腺素和多巴胺在死亡率方面没有显著差异。目前研究表明,应用去甲肾上腺素可以降低心源性和感染性休克患者的死亡率(*Ann Emerg Med*, 2013, 61: 351)。

 87. 去甲肾上腺素和脓毒性休克

Norepinephrine is considered the vasopressor of first choice for septic shock. Why is phenylephrine not recommended for use in the treatment of most cases of septic shock?

去甲肾上腺素被认为是脓毒性休克的首选升压药。为什么不建议在治疗脓毒性休克时使用去氧肾上腺素?

Phenylephrine, a pure alpha-adrenergic agonist, can decrease stroke volume and is not recommended for use in septic shock except in very specific circumstances (e. g. cardiac output is known to be high and BP low).

去氧肾上腺素，一个纯 α 肾上腺素受体兴奋药，可以减少心脏每搏排血量，因此不建议在脓毒性休克时应用，除非极特殊的情况（如心排血量高时血压仍然处于较低的状态）(*Ann Emerg Med*, 2014, 63: 35)。

 ## 88. 激素在脓毒性休克中的作用

The use of empiric corticosteroid administration is not recommended for all patients with shock. When should the use of low-dose hydrocortisone be considered?

所有休克患者常规使用皮质类固醇已不再被推荐使用。什么时候可以考虑使用低剂量氢化可的松？

For adult patients with septic shock, hydrocortisone should be considered only in cases of persistent hemodynamic instability (i. e. the patient fails to respond to IV fluid and vasopressor therapy).

成人脓毒性休克患者，只有在顽固性血流动力学不稳定的情况下（即患者对静脉补液和升压药治疗无反应）才可考虑使用氢化可的松(*Ann Emerg Med*, 2014, 64: 35)。

 ## 89. 弥散性血管内凝血的实验室指标

A clinical diagnosis of disseminated intravascular coagulation (DIC) is based on consistent clinical presentation coupled with laboratory results. What lab results suggest DIC?

弥散性血管内凝血(DIC)的临床诊断要根据明确的临床表现，结合实验室结果才能确定，哪些实验室结果提示 DIC？

Lowplatelets elevated fibrin-related marker (eg. fibrin degradation products), elevated PT, and low fibrinogen level. However, the fibrinogen level may be elevated as an acute-phase reactant. D-dimer is usually high.

血小板减低，纤维蛋白升高相关的标记（如纤维蛋白降解产物），凝血酶原时间(PT)升高, 和纤维蛋白原水平降低。然而, 纤维蛋白原水平可能作为一种急性期反应物升高。D - 二聚体通常是增高的 (*Mayo Clin Proc*, 2012, 87:799)。

90. 体外膜氧合(ECMO)在严重哮喘抢救中的应用

In exceedingly rare circumstances, aggressive treatment for acute respiratory failure due to severe asthma will not provide adequate gas exchange. What next step should the clinician consider?

极为罕见的情况下, 由于严重哮喘引起的急性呼吸衰竭经积极治疗后, 仍不能提供足够的气体交换, 临床医生下一步应该考虑做什么呢?

Case reports describe successful use of extracorporeal membrane oxygenation in adult and pediatric patients with severe asthma after other aggressive measures have failed to reverse hypoxemia and hypercarbia.

有成功病例报告, 患有严重哮喘的成人和儿童经其他积极的措施都未能扭转低氧血症和高碳酸血症时, 可使用体外膜肺氧合(ECMO)(*Circulation*, 2010, 122:S829)。

91. 正常人无氧多久后氧才降到90%以下?

If a healthy adult is preoxygenated with 100% oxygen and ventilating effectively and then becomes apneic, how long will it take before oxygen saturation decreases to less than 90%?

如果一个健康的成年人在用100%氧有效氧合和通气后, 出现呼吸暂停, 在无继续给氧的条件下, 大概会需要多长时间氧饱和度会降到90%以下?

6 minutes.

6分钟 (*Ann Emerg Med*, 2008, 52:3)。

92. 琥珀胆碱与钾

In individuals without any neuromuscular disease, succinylcholine typically produces a transient rise in serum potassium of how much? In patients with neuromuscular disease?

在没有任何神经肌肉疾病的患者中，琥珀胆碱通常会使血钾短暂升高多少？在有神经肌肉疾病的患者中又怎样？

In individuals without neuromuscular disease, succinylcholine typically produces a transient rise in serum potassium of approximately 0.55 mEq/L. Patients with neuromuscular disease experience an average increase in of 1.8 mEq/L.

在无神经肌肉疾病的个体患者中，琥珀胆碱通常会使钾短暂升高大约 0.55 mEq/L。而在患有神经肌肉疾病的患者中，平均钾增高值为 1.8 mEq/L(*J Emerg Med*, 2012, 43: 280)。

 93. 如何计算罗库溴铵的剂量？

Succinylcholine dosing is based on total body weight. What about rocuronium dosing? Why does it matter?

琥珀胆碱的剂量是按身体总重量计算的。罗库溴铵的剂量是如何计算的？有什么关系呢？

Rocuronium dosing typically is based on ideal body weight. A recent clinical study showed that dosing by total body weight can increase duration of action by up to 50%.

罗库溴铵剂量通常是根据理想体重计算的。最近的临床研究表明，按身体总重量计算的药量将使作用时间延长 50% (*Can J Anaesth*, 2013, 60: 552)。

94. 氯胺酮的两个绝对禁忌证

What are the 2 absolute contraindications to ketamine use for ED procedures?

急诊操作时使用氯胺酮镇静的两个绝对禁忌证是什么?

Age <3 months and known or suspected schizophrenia.

年龄 <3 个月和已知或怀疑患有精神分裂症者(*Ann Emerg Med*, 2013, 57: 449)。

95. 3 岁以下的儿童不能长时间用异丙酚

Why should propofol not be used for long-term sedation in children younger than 3 years?

为什么对 3 岁以下的儿童不能长时间用异丙酚镇静?

Propofol should not be used for long-term sedation in children <3 years because of the reported association with fatal metabolic acidosis.

3 岁以下的儿童不能长时间用异丙酚镇静,因其长期应用可导致有生命危险的代谢性酸中毒(*Crit Care Med*, 2013, 41: 580)。

96. 低温时出现心房颤动的处理

You are caring for a patient in the ED who is quite hypothermic (87℉) after having been found on a sidewalk in the middle of winter. Are you concerned that the patient is found to be in atrial fibrillation?

深冬季节,你在急诊科抢救一个在人行道上被发现的相当低温的患者(T30.6℃)。如患者出现心房颤动,你应如何处理?

Atrial fibrillation is common when the core temperature is less than 90 °F and is not worrisome in the absence of other signs of cardiac instability。

心房颤动在中心温度低于32℃时是常见的，但在没有心脏不稳定迹象时，不需要太担心（*N Engl J Med*，2012，367：1930）。

97. 冻僵与体外肺膜氧合

Which patients with accidental hypothermia should be transported by EMS directly to a center capable of providing extracorporeal membrane oxygenation or cardiopulmonary bypass?

哪些意外性低温（冻僵）的患者应通过医疗急救系统（EMS）直接转运到一个能够提供体外肺膜氧合或体外循环的中心？

Patients with prehospital cardiac instability (e. g. , SBP < 90 mmHg or ventricular arrhythmias), those with a core temperature < (82 °F) and those in cardiac arrest.

院前心脏功能不稳定的患者（例如收缩压 < 90 mmHg 或有室性心律失常），中心温度低于（27.8℃）和心脏骤停的患者（*N Engl J Med*，2012，367：1930）。

98. 抗精神病药恶性综合征

How does neuroleptic malignant syndrome (NMS) present clinically?

抗精神病药恶性综合征（NMS）的典型临床表现是什么？

NMS is characterized by hyperthermia, autonomic instability, neuromuscular rigidity, and altered mental status. Temperatures average 103 °F. It is often difficult to distinguish from serotonin syndrome.

抗精神病药恶性综合征（NMS）的临床特点有高热，自主神经失调，神经肌肉强直，神志异常。平均体温为 39.4℃。它往往与 5 - 羟色胺综合征难以区分（*J Emerg Med*，2013，43：906）。

讨论：抗精神病药恶性综合征与 5 - 羟色胺综合征的区别

		抗精神病药恶性综合征	5 - 羟色胺综合征
诱发因素		多巴胺拮抗药	5 - 羟色胺能药物
发作时间		1 ~ 3 天	< 12 小时
相同点	生命体征	血压高 心率快 呼吸急促 体温高（ > 40℃ ）	血压高 心率快 呼吸急促 体温高（ > 40℃ ）
	黏膜	唾液分泌亢进	唾液分泌亢进
类似点	皮肤	大汗 苍白	大汗
	神志	异常	异常
	肌肉	所有肌肉僵直（铅管症）	张力增加，尤其是下肢
特异点	各种反射	低	亢进，痉挛
	瞳孔	正常	扩大
	肠鸣音	正常或减低	亢进

 99. 五羟色胺综合征症状的持续时间

Typically, symptoms of the serotonin syndrome resolve how long after discontinuation of the offending agent?

通常情况下，五羟色胺综合征的症状在停用致病药物后多久消失？

Generally, symptoms of the serotonin syndrome resolve 24 – 48 hours after discontinuation of the offending agent. If symptoms persist beyond 72 hours, alternative diagnoses should be sought.

一般情况下，五羟色胺综合征的症状在停用致病药物后 24 ~ 48 小时内缓解。如果症状持续超过 72 小时，则应寻找其他诊断（ *N Engl J Med*，2013，369：1930）。

100. 超声测量下腔静脉直径

Recently, the ultrasonographic measurement of the diameter of IVC to detect hypovolemia has become popular. Why does the dIVC reflect volume status more closely than other parameters based on the arterial system, such as BP and heart rate?

最近，用超声测量下腔静脉的直径来判断血容量不足已被广泛接受。为什么下腔静脉直径反映容量状态要比其他参数，如反映动脉系统的血压和心率更加敏感和准确？

The dIVC has not been found to be affected by the body's compensatory vasoconstrictor response to volume loss. Hence, it reflects volume status more closely than other parameters based on the arterial system.

下腔静脉直径并不受到机体对容量损失所产生的代偿性血管收缩反应的影响。因此，它反映容量状态要比其他反映动脉系统的指标更加敏感和准确（*J Emerg Med*, 2013, 45: 592)。

 101. 中心静脉导管的位置

An appropriately placed central venous catheter should terminate in the SVC, at the level of what landmark on chest x-ray?

放置合适的中心静脉导管应终止于 SVC，但在胸部 X 线片上所显示导管的标准位置是什么？

The central venous catheter should terminate approximately at the level of the right tracheobronchial angle (Broder, Diagnostic Imaging for the Emergency Physician, 2011).

中心静脉导管的管端在胸部 X 线片上所显示的位置应终止在右侧气管/支气管角的水平(*Diagnostic Imaging for the Emergency Physician. Broder. ed*, 2011)。

102. 短暂性脑缺血发作后的脑卒中发生率

What is the risk of stroke during the 3 months after a transient ischemic attack?

短暂性脑缺血(TIA)发作后3个月内发生脑卒中的风险是多少?

The risk of stroke during the 3 months after a TIA has been estimated to be approximately 10%, with half of these strokes occurring within the first 2 days.

短暂性脑缺血(TIA)后3个月内发生脑卒中的风险已被预测为10%，这些脑卒中的一半在TIA发生后的2天内发生 (*Ann Emerg Med*, 2013, 57: 14)。

 # 103. 脑灰质与白质分界丧失的意义

What is the significance of the finding of loss of gray-white differentiation on noncontrast CT of the head?

在头部CT平扫影像上，脑灰质与白质分界丧失(图21)的意义是什么?

It is a significant early sign of cerebral ischemia, occurring within the first few hours after symptom onset, because there is an increase in the relative water concentration of ischemic tissues.

这是一个显著的脑缺血早期表现，通常在症状发作后的几个小时内出现，原因是由于缺血组织内相对水浓度的增加(*Stroke*, 2009, 40: 3646)。

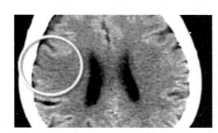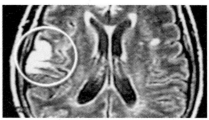

图21　脑灰质与白质与界丧失

104. CT 平扫诊断后颅窝脑卒中

Non-contrast computed tomography is particularly poor at detecting strokes in the posterior fossa, compared with its ability to diagnose acute supratentorial ischemia. Why?

与诊断急性幕上脑缺血的敏感度相比，计算机断层（CT）平扫在诊断后颅窝脑卒中时的敏感性是特别差的。为什么呢？

Because of the presence of beam-hardening artifact due to the amount of bone locally, as well as the relative time delay for strokes to appear on neuroimaging in the white matter relative to the gray matter.

是因为有局部骨质强度所造成的射束硬化伪影（BHA）的影响，另外在神经影像上脑白质的脑卒中病变通常要比脑灰质的病变出现的晚（*J Emerg Med*，2012，42：559）。

 105. 基底动脉闭塞

Sudden, unexplained nontraumatic comas is not an uncommon ED issue. Recently, the addition of CTA to a standard noncontrast CT has been recommended. This approach would diagnose what important condition that warrants emergent treatment?

不明原因的非创伤性昏迷在急诊科还是比较常见的。最近，除了一个标准的CT平扫，还建议使用CTA（CT血管造影）。这种方法将诊断出一个什么需要紧急处理的情况？

Basilar artery occlusion; specific treatment, such as IV thrombolysis or endovascular treatment, improve outcomes with an average 50% of good neurologic outcomes at 3 months, whereas 90% of patients who did not receive therapy died.

基底动脉闭塞。特异的治疗，如静脉溶栓或血管内介入，可改善患者的预后，使平均50%的人在3个月内有良好的神经系统的恢复，而90%没有接受治疗的患者将死亡（*J Emerg Med*，2012，43：e265）。

106. 脑卒中发作后 24 至 48 小时内的病情变化

What portion of patients have neurological worsening during the first 24 to 48 hours after acute stroke?

急性脑卒中发作后 24 至 48 小时内，多大一部分患者会有病情恶化？

Approximately 25% of patients may have neurological worsening during the first 24 to 48 hours after stroke, and it is difficult to predict which patients will deteriorate.

在最初 24 至 48 小时内，约 25% 的患者可能会出现神经系统病情恶化，并且很难预测哪些患者会恶化（*Stroke*, 2013, 44: 870）。

107. 急性脑卒中时的 QT 间期延长

QT prolongation is commonly seen in acute stroke. Although the pathogenesis not well understood, what is felt to be the underlying cause?

急性脑卒中常出现 QT 间期延长。虽然其发病机制还不是很清楚，有可能会是什么原因？

Sympathetic hyperactivity during the acute stage of cerebral infarction is considered to be associated with QT interval prolongation in acute stroke populations and has a positive correlation with size of infarction.

急性期脑梗死的交感神经功能亢进被认为与急性脑卒中人群中 QT 间期延长有关，同时与梗死面积呈正相关（*Am J Emerg Med*, 2013, 31: 1719. e5）。

108. 接受组织纤溶酶原激活剂治疗的患者都患有缺血性脑卒中吗?

According to available literature, of patients who receive tissue plasminogen activator for acute stroke, what portion turned out to have a stroke mimic? What portion does not develop ischemic injury and are diagnosed as having TIA?

根据现有的文献,在接受组织纤溶酶原激活剂(tPA)的急性脑卒中患者中,会有多少患者实际上是患有脑卒中类似症状? 多少患者不会出现缺血性脑损伤,而被诊断为短暂性脑缺血发作(TIA)?

A retrospective analysis of 254 patients who received tPA showed that 3.5% had a stroke mimic. Another 9% did not develop ischemic injury and were diagnosed as having TIA, and 87% had ischemic stroke.

一个254例接受tPA后患者的回顾性分析表明,3.5%患有脑卒中类似症状。另外9%的患者并未造成缺血性脑损伤,而被诊断为短暂性脑缺血发作(TIA),剩下的87%为缺血性脑卒中(*Am J Emerg Med*, 2012, 30: 794)。

109. 组织纤溶酶原激活剂与血管性水肿

An estimated 5% of patients treated with tPA for acute ischemic stroke develop angioedema. Why would you not expect antihistamines and glucocorticoids to be of significant help?

估计有5%的急性缺血性脑卒中患者在接受组织纤溶酶原激活剂(tPA)治疗后出现血管性水肿。为什么你不期待使用抗组胺药和糖皮质激素会有显著的帮助?

tPA causes plasmin-mediated bradykinin release whereas antihistamines andglucocorticoids are targeted toward mast cell-mediated angioedema.

组织纤溶酶原激活剂(tPA)引起的血管性水肿是由纤维蛋白溶酶介导的缓激肽释放增加所致,而抗组胺药和糖皮质激素对由肥大细胞介导的血管性水肿有效(*J Emerg Med*, 2013, 45: 789)。

110. 缺血性脑卒中后行去骨瓣减压术

What is the purpose of decompressive hemicraniectomy (temporary removal of a large part of the skull) for large space-occupying middle-cerebral-artery ischemic cerebral infarcts?

大面积占位性大脑中动脉缺血性脑梗死后行去骨瓣减压术(临时去除颅骨的一大部分)的目的是什么?

Large space-occupying MCA infarcts are associated with the development of massive brain edema. Decompressive hemicraniectomy allows edematous tissue to expand outside the neurocranium, thereby preventing fatal herniation.

大面积占位性大脑中动脉缺血性脑梗死会导致严重的脑水肿。去骨瓣减压术可以使水肿的脑组织扩大到颅外，从而防止致死性脑疝形成(*N Engl J Med*, 2014, 370: 1091)。

111. 颈动脉内膜切除术应在何时进行？

A patient presents to the ED with an ischemic stroke or a TIA in the carotid-artery distribution. If a carotid artery stenosis is identified, when should carotid endarterectomy be performed?

一个患者因颈动脉分布区域的缺血性脑卒中或短暂性脑缺血发作到急诊科就诊。如果诊断为颈动脉狭窄，那么颈动脉内膜切除术应在何时进行？

In patients with an ischemic stroke or a TIA in the carotid-artery distribution, carotid endarterectomy should be considered within 2 weeks if there is stenosis of > 70% of the diameter of the ipsilateral carotid artery.

对于颈动脉分布区域的缺血性脑卒中或短暂性脑缺血发作的患者，如果同侧颈动脉的直径狭窄 >70%，颈动脉内膜切除术需要在 2 个星期内进行(*N Engl J Med*, 2013, 369: 1143)。

112. 非外伤性脑血肿扩张

How common is hematoma expansion of a spontaneous, nontraumatic intracerebral hemorrhage following initial CT scan?

在初始 CT 扫描后，一个非外伤性脑出血的血肿扩大是常见的，比例如何？

Among patients undergoing head CT within 3 hours of ICH onset, 28% – 38% have hematoma expansion of >1/3 on follow-up CT. Hematoma expansion is predictive of clinical deterioration and increased morbidity and mortality.

患脑出血(ICH)的患者在就诊 3 小时内重复行脑 CT 检查，将会发现 28% ~ 38% 的患者血肿会增加至少 1/3。血肿扩大是一个预测临床恶化、发病率和死亡率增加的指标（*Stroke*, 2010, 41: 2108）。

113. 脑出血的功能恢复

Intracerebral hemorrhage is one of the most devastating forms of stroke. what portion of patients achieve functional independence?

脑出血(ICH)是脑卒中最危险的形式。有多少患者能恢复到功能独立的状态？

The median 1 – month case fatality rate for ICH is 40%, and only 12 – 39% of patients achieve functional independence.

1 个月内脑出血(ICH)的死亡率中位数为 40%，并且只有 12% ~ 39% 的患者可以恢复功能独立的状态（*N Engl J Med*, 2013, 368: 2426）。

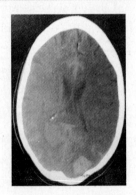

图 22　脑出血

114. 动脉瘤性蛛网膜下隙出血

Most intracranial aneurysms remain asymptomatic until they rupture. Do most aneurysmal subarachnoid hemorrhages occur during physical exertion or stress?

大多数颅内动脉瘤在破裂之前都无症状。多数的动脉瘤性蛛网膜下隙出血（ASAH）会在身体活动或精神压力下发生吗？

ASAH can occur during exertion or stress, but in a review of 513 patients with ASAH, the highest incidence of rupture occurred while patients were engaged in their daily routines, in the absence of strenuous physical activity.

动脉瘤性蛛网膜下隙出血（ASAH）可在劳累或紧张时发生。但在一个513例ASAH的评估文献中，破裂发生频率最高的是患者在进行日常活动并没有强烈的体力活动时（*Stroke*, 2012, 43: 1463）。

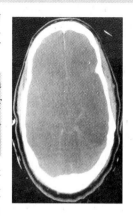

图23 蛛网膜下隙出血

 115. 脑脊液黄染的意义

Xanthochromia is a yellow discoloration of the CSF supernatant that results from the breakdown of RBCs into oxyhemoglobin, methemoglobin, and bilirubin. Why is its presence in CSF more specific for SAH than the presence of RBC?

脑脊液（CSF）黄染是指CSF的上清液呈黄色，它来自于破裂的红细胞中的含氧血红蛋白、高铁血红蛋白、胆红素。为什么脑脊液中脑脊液黄染要比红细胞的存在对诊断蛛网膜下隙出血（SAH）更特异？

Because xanthochromia is the result of a process that only occurs in vivo, its presence is more specific for SAH than the presence of RBCs.

由于黄变是唯一能够在体内发生的过程，在蛛网膜下隙出血（SAH）中它的存在比红细胞存在更特异（*J Emerg Med*，2010，39：13）。

116. CT 诊断蛛网膜下隙出血的限制

What might explain why uenhanced head CT is more sensitive for subarachnoid hemorrhage when performed sooner following headache onset?

为什么头颅 CT 平扫在由蛛网膜下隙出血引起头痛的患者中发病后越早做越敏感？

A relatively small volume of blood released into the subarachnoid space will diffuse away from the source of bleeding and hemolyze within hours, rendering CT less able to distinguish the blood from CSF as time passes.

体积相对较小的血液释放进入蛛网膜下隙将扩散至远离出血源的地方，并在几小时内发生溶血，因此随着时间的推移，CT 鉴别血液和脑脊液的能力也随之下降（*British Med J*，2011，343：4277）。

117. CT 诊断贫血患者的急性蛛网膜下隙出血

How does the presence of anemia affect the ability of CT scan to detect acute subarachnoid hemorrhage?

贫血的存在会如何影响 CT 扫描诊断急性蛛网膜下隙出血？

Intracranial blood in anemic patients (Hct <30%) may appear isodense with brain and therefore more difficult to see and can result in falsely-negative CT for SAH.

贫血患者（血细胞比容，Hct <30%）的颅内血肿可能会呈现与脑组织一样的密度，因此更难以发现出血，容易造成 CT 在诊断蛛网膜下隙出血时的假阴性（*J Emerg Med*，2008，34：237）。

118. 蛛网膜下隙出血后脑血管痉挛出现的时间

Cerebral vasospasm may occur when cerebral vessels are exposed to blood in the subarachnoid space. Cerebral vasospasm is one of the leading causes of morbi-mortality following aneurysmal SAH. When does cerebral vasospasm typically occur after SAH?

脑血管痉挛可能是由蛛网膜下隙的血接触并刺激脑血管产生。脑血管痉挛是动脉瘤性蛛网膜下隙出血(ASAH)后出现并发症和死亡的主要原因之一。在蛛网膜下隙出血(SAH)后脑血管痉挛通常会在什么时间内出现?

It typically occurs 4 – 14 days after the SAH, with a peak incidence between 6 and 10 days.

它通常发生蛛网膜下隙出血(SAH)后的 4 ~ 14 天,发病高峰在 6 天到 10 天之间(*Intervent Neurol*,2013,2:30)。

119. 蛛网膜下隙出血导致血管痉挛的处理

Patients with subarachnoid hemorrhage are at risk of developing delayed cerebral ischemia as a result of arterial vasospasm. How to manage this?

蛛网膜下隙出血患者会由于动脉血管痉挛导致迟发性脑缺血。应如何处理这一现象?

Vasospasm most commonly occurs 1 week after SAH; it is a major cause of morbidity. Management involves maintenance of cerebral perfusion by establishing euvolemia and considering induced hypertension after the aneurysm is secured.

血管痉挛最常发生在蛛网膜下隙出血(SAH)1 周后,它是造成合并症的主要原因。处理主要是通过液体平衡维持脑灌注并考虑在血管瘤稳定后适当升高血压(*Ann Emerg Med*,2014,64:248)。

讨论:蛛网膜下隙出血后脑血管痉挛

1. 脑血管痉挛发生在70%的蛛网膜下隙出血患者中，其中30%的患者需要治疗。

2. 其症状包括肢体肌力降低，神志改变，烦躁等。

3. 治疗可给予尼卡地平（nicardipine）和3H方案（适当升高血压，扩容和血液稀释）。

 120. 第一次癫痫发作是否需要使用抗癫痫药?

Emergency Physicians often encounter patients having experienced a first-time seizure and must make decisions about the initiation of anticonvulsant therapy. After a single seizure, what portion of patients will have a recurrence within 2 years?

急诊医师经常会遇到第一次癫痫发作的患者，必须决定是否需要开始进行抗癫痫治疗。在仅仅一次发作后，将有多少比例的患者会在2年内复发?

About 25% will have a recurrence within 2 years in the absence of factors that predict a high probability of recurrence (e. g. , epileptiform activity detected on an EEG or a known cause such as remote major head trauma).

在没有预测高复发危险因素的情况下（如脑电图显示癫痫样活动或已知既往头部外伤史），大概有25%的患者会在2年内复发（*N Engl J Med*, 2008, 359: 166）。

 121. 乳酸水平在癫痫发作中的作用

Seizures can result in a profound elevation of lactate levels, which is transient; once the seizure has resolved, lactate production ceases, and lactate is rapidlycleared. Lactate levels are expected to remain elevated for how long after a seizure?

癫痫发作可以导致明显的乳酸水平增高，但这是短暂的;一旦癫痫停止，乳酸产生随即停止，并被迅速清除。乳酸水平在癫痫发作后会持续升高多久?

Persistently elevated lactate levels beyond the expected 1 to 2 hours after a seizure may suggest a different or concomitant underlying etiology and warrant further consideration.

如果在癫痫发作停止 1 ~ 2 小时后乳酸水平持续升高，要考虑不同的或同时存在的原因，需要作进一步的评估（*Mayo Clin Proc*，2012，88：1127）。

122. 乙醇引起的癫痫的发作时间

When do alcohol-related seizures typically occur after the last drink? Multiple seizures occur in 60% of patients without treatment; what is the usual interval between the first and the last seizure?

由乙醇引起的癫痫通常是在最后一次饮酒后多长时间发生？60% 未经治疗的患者会出现多次发作，第一次和最后一次发作的间隔通常是多久？

Alcohol-related seizures occur 6 – 48 hrs after the last drink. When multiple seizures occur, the interval between the first and the last seizure is usually less than 6 hrs.

乙醇引起的癫痫发生在最后一次饮酒后的 6 ~ 48 小时。当多次癫痫发生时，第一次和最后的发作之间的间隔通常短于 6 小时（*J Emerg Med*，2006，31：157）。

123. 成人细菌性脑膜炎

If a stable adult patient has meningitis symptoms for greater than 48 hours, is bacterial meningitis excluded with reasonable certainty?

如果一个稳定的成年脑膜炎患者的症状超过 48 小时，那么有明确理由排除细菌性脑膜炎吗？

No. Approximately 50% of adult bacterial meningitis patients have a symptom duration of greater than 24 hours.

没有。约 50% 的成人细菌性脑膜炎患者的症状持续时间超过 24 小时（*Ann Emerg Med*，2012，56：227）。

124. 医源性细菌性脑膜炎

Iatrogenic bacterial meningitis is a serious complication of neuraxial procedures, such as spinal and epidural anesthesia or LP. What is the source of infection in cases of IBM? (hint: it is not the patient's skin)

医源性细菌性脑膜炎(IBM)是一种由椎管内操作产生的严重并发症,如脊髓或硬膜外麻醉或腰椎穿刺。IBM 感染的来源是什么?(提示:不是患者的皮肤)

Evidence strongly points to droplets from the mouth or upper airway of medical personnel as the source of infection in cases of IBM.

有明确证据显示医务人员口腔或上呼吸道飞沫颗粒是 IBM 的传染源(*Can J Emerg Med*, 2012, 14: 259)。

125. 腰椎穿刺与脑膜炎

Can meningitis develop after lumbar puncture?

腰椎穿刺(LP)后会感染脑膜炎吗?

Meningitis develops after LP in approximately 1 in 50,000 cases, with about 80 cases reported annually in the US. The majority of cases occur after spinal anesthesia or myelography.

腰椎穿刺(LP)后发生脑膜炎的比例大约在 1:50,000,美国每年报道约 80 例。大多数病例出现在腰麻或脊髓造影后(*N Engl J Med*, 2010, 362: 146)。

126. 口服抗生素对脑脊液分析的影响

When considering the possibility of bacterial meningitis in a child in the ED, how does recent treatment with oral antibiotics affect CSF analysis and interpretation in making this diagnosis?

在急诊科考虑一个儿童患细菌性脑膜炎的可能性时，近期口服抗生素对脑脊液（CSF）的检查和解释有何影响？

Multiple studies have shown that in most cases, treatment with oral antibiotics prior to CSF analysis does not alter underlying abnormalities in CSF composition so as to obscure the diagnosis of meningitis.

多项研究表明，大多数情况下，在进行脑脊液（CSF）检查前口服抗生素治疗并不改变 CSF 相关的异常成分，因此不会影响脑膜炎的诊断（*J Emerg Med*，2014，46：141）。

 127. 与脑膜炎球菌病患者密切接触的定义

The CDC recommends postexposure prophylaxis for close contacts of patients with meningococcal disease. What defines a close contact?

CDC 建议与脑膜炎球菌病患者密切接触后要预防性用药。如何定义密切接触？

①household members；②child-care center personnel；③persons directly exposed to the patient's oral secretions（e. g., by kissing, mouth-to-mouth resuscitation, endotracheal intubation, or endotracheal tube management）.

家庭成员；幼儿园工作人员；患者口腔分泌物直接接触者（如通过接吻，口对口人工呼吸，气管插管或气管插管管理人员）（*MMWR Weekly*，2010，59：1480）。

第
五
篇

神
经
系
统
疾
病
篇

128. 为什么腰椎穿刺后脑脊液要立即分析？

With a traumatic LP, the centrifuged CSF supernatant should be crystal clear; with subarachnoid hemorrhage, the tainted centrifuged supernatant is xanthochromic. Why must the CSF be analyzed immediately post-LP for this distinction to be valid?

创伤性腰椎穿刺（LP）获得的脑脊液（CSF），经离心后的悬浮液应该是清澈的；蛛网膜下隙出血患者的脑脊液离心后，其悬浮液呈黄色。为什么这种区别一定要在 LP 后立即对脑脊液进行分析才是有效的？

With traumatic LP, the centrifuged CSF supernatant is clear because the blood is freshly arrived and RBC membrane intact. Lysis of CSF RBCs starts after about 4 hrs, so it is important that the CSF is analyzed immediately post-LP.

创伤性腰椎穿刺（LP）所获得的脑脊液（CSF）经离心后，其悬浮液是清澈的，因为新鲜血液的红细胞膜完好。脑脊液中红细胞裂解约在 4 小时后发生。因此，LP 后立即对脑脊液进行分析是重要的（*J Emerg Med*, 2014, 46: 141）。

 129. 腰椎穿刺后脑脊液的恢复

The CSF fills the subarachnoid space. An adult produces approximately 500 mL of CSF daily, at a rate of about 0.5 mL/min. How long does it take to reconstitute the typical volume removed by a routine lumbar puncture (3 – 5 mL)?

脑脊液（CSF）填充蛛网膜下隙。一个成年人以约 0.5 mL/min 的速率每天产生 500 mL CSF。在常规腰椎穿刺（LP）后多久可以恢复抽出的 CSF（3~5 mL）？

The volume removed by a routine LP is reconstituted in <1 hr.

常规 LP 取出的 CSF 容量会在 1 小时内恢复（*J Emerg Med*, 2014, 46: 141）。

130. 假性脑瘤与腰椎穿刺

The most serious complication of an LP is cerebral herniation, which is ascribed to rapid CSF extraction when there is increased ICP. Pseudotumor cerebri is characterized by increased ICP, yet is diagnosed via LP. Why is an LP safe in this setting?

腰椎穿刺(LP)的一个最严重的并发症是脑疝,这是由于在颅内压(ICP)升高时快速提取脑脊液所致。假性脑瘤的 ICP 都高,其诊断要通过 LP。为什么此时的 LP 是安全的?

Herniation results from rapid CSF extraction when there is raised ICP with an abnormal pressure gradient. In pseudotumor cerebri, there is uniformly raised ICP within the entire CNS so there is no pressure gradient and LP is safe.

快速抽取脑脊液发生脑疝是在 ICP 升高的同时还要有异常的压力差。假性脑瘤是在整个中枢神经系统内 ICP 均匀升高,不存在压力差的问题,因此 LP 是安全的(*J Emerg Med*, 2014, 46: 141)。

131. 垂体卒中

What is pituitary apoplexy?

什么是垂体卒中?

Pituitary apoplexy is hemorrhage or infarction of the pituitary gland. It occurs most commonly in patients with pituitary macroadenomas but can occur in pregnancy, general anesthesia, and bromocriptine therapy.

垂体卒中是指垂体内出血或梗死,它最常出现于垂体大腺瘤患者,但也可在妊娠、全身麻醉和应用溴隐亭时发生(*Mayo Clin Proc*, 2010, 85: e44)。

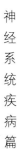

132. 快速一次注射葡萄糖会加重韦尼克脑病吗?

It is sometimes stated that a single acute administration of glucose can precipitate Wernicke's encephalopathy. Is this true?

有人说,快速一次注射葡萄糖会加重韦尼克脑病。这是真的吗?

Wernicke's encephalopathy can occur with prolonged glucose or carbohydrate loading in the absence of thiamine. However, a single acute administration of glucose does not appear to cause this effect.

韦尼克脑病可发生在缺乏硫胺素情况下长时间葡萄糖或糖类物(碳水化合物)超负荷。然而,快速一次注射葡萄糖不会有什么影响(*Ann Emerg Med*,2007,50:715)。

 133. 静脉窦血栓形成的三联征

What is the classic clinical triad of dural sinus thrombosis (DST)?

什么是典型的静脉窦血栓三联征(DST)?

The classic triad of DST is headache, papilledema, and high CSF opening pressure. MRI with magnetic resonance venography is considered the gold standard for diagnosis.

静脉窦血栓三联征(DST)的典型症状是头痛、视乳头水肿、脑脊液初始压力高。磁共振成像与磁共振静脉造影被认为是诊断 DST 的金标准(*Am J Emerg Med*,2007,25:218)。

134. 格林 – 巴利综合征(GBS)的潜伏期

When do symptoms of Guillain-Barré syndrome typically occur after a febrile illness?

格林 – 巴利综合征(GBS)的症状通常在发热性疾病之后多久出现?

Symptoms of GBS most commonly occur 2 to 4 weeks after a febrile illness; however, it can present up to 12 weeks with cases of Campylobacter jejuni.

格林 – 巴利综合征(GBS)的症状最常在发热性疾病后 2~4 周出现,但是在空肠弯曲菌感染时,这个时间长达 12 周(*Am J Emerg Med*, 2014, 32:110. e5)。

135. 腰椎穿刺对格林 – 巴利综合征的诊断价值

A patient presents to the ED with progressive bilateral and symmetric weakness of the legs, and Guillain – Barré syndrome is suspected. Is an LP typically diagnostic?

一个因进行性对称性双下肢无力到急诊就诊的患者,你怀疑格林 – 巴利综合征(GBS)。腰椎穿刺(LP)具有确切的诊断价值吗?

An LP is performed primarily to rule out other diagnoses (e. g. Lyme disease). A misconception is that there should always be albuminocytologic dissociation; this is present in no more than 50% of GBS cases during the 1st week.

腰椎穿刺(LP)主要是为了排除其他疾病的诊断(如莱姆病)。一定要有蛋白细胞分离是一个误解,因为在第 1 周只有不到 50% 的格林 – 巴利综合征(GBS)患者有此现象(*N Engl J Med*, 2012, 366:2294)。

136. 上行性肌无力

What electrolyte abnormality can produce an ascending muscle weakness that begins with the legs and progresses to the trunk and arms, mimicking Guillain-Barre syndrome?

哪种电解质异常可以产生类似于格林 - 巴利综合征从腿到躯干和手臂的上行性肌肉无力?

Severe hypokalemia (< 2. 5 mEq/L) can also produce ascending muscle weakness.

严重低钾血症(<2.5 mEq/L), 也可以产生上行性肌肉无力(*Ann Emerg Med*, 2013, 62: S129)。

 137. 低钾性周期性麻痹患者的饮食

Why must a patient with a history of hypokalemic periodic paralysis avoid meals heavy in carbohydrates?

为什么低钾性周期性麻痹患者必须避免食用过量的糖类物(碳水化合物)?

Consumption of large amounts of carbohydrate increases serum insulin which drives potassium into the muscle cells. In patients with periodic paralysis, a genetic mutation allows excessive amounts of potassium enter the muscle cell.

食用大量的糖类物(碳水化合物)会增加胰岛素分泌, 胰岛素将会驱使钾进入到肌肉细胞内(使血清钾进一步降低)。周期性麻痹的患者, 基因突变使过量的钾进入肌肉细胞(*J Emerg Med*, 2009, 36: 236)。

讨论: 低钾性周期性麻痹患者的饮食

高蛋白饮食, 避免高糖类物(碳水化合物)和高盐, 注意补钾(6 支香蕉相当于 72mEq 的钾)。同时要避免剧烈运动。

138. 闭锁综合征

Locked-in syndrome is the combination of quadriplegia and anarthria (inability to speak), with the preservation of consciousness. What is the cause of most cases?

闭锁综合征(Locked-in syndrome)是四肢瘫伴构音障碍(不能说话)的一种综合征,但意识清楚。大多数情况下,是由什么原因引起的?

The majority of cases are caused by basilarartery occlusion leading to brainstem infarction in the ventral pons.

大多数情况下是由基底动脉梗死导致中脑腹侧脑干梗死引起(*Can J Emerg Med*, 2012, 14: 317)。

139. 短暂性全面遗忘症

Transient global amnesia is characterized by the sudden onset of dense anterograde amnesia, without alteration consciousness or focal neurologic deficits or seizure activity. What are the proposed theories regarding the pathophysiology of TGA?

短暂性全面遗忘症(TGA)的特点是突然发作的强烈的前瞻性遗忘,没有意识改变或局部性神经功能缺损或癫痫发作。TGA 在病理生理方面的发生机制是什么?

Theories to explain TGA include migraine, seizure, arterial ischemia, and venous congestion of the brain leading to ischemia, but the precise mechanisms remain unclear.

产生短暂性全面遗忘证(TGA)的可能机制包括偏头痛、癫痫发作、动脉缺血、脑静脉充血导致的脑缺血,但确切的发病机制尚不清楚 (*J Emerg Med*, 2011, 41: 267)。

第五篇 神经系统疾病篇

140. Ramsay Hunt 综合征

Ramsay Hunt Syndrome is a peripheral facial nerve palsy accompanied by a vesicular rash on the ear (herpes zoster oticus). Although similar to Bell's palsy, what are the important differences clinically?

Ramsay Hunt 综合征（RHS）是一种周围性面神经瘫痪并在耳朵上有水疱样皮疹（耳带状疱疹）。虽然类似于贝尔麻痹，临床上它们之间的重要区别是什么？

RHS, although similar to Bell's palsy, is often more severe, with a higher likelihood of permanent sequelae and multiple cranial nerve involvement.

Ramsay Hunt 综合征（RHS），虽然类似于贝尔麻痹，但病情常常是更严重的，发生永久性后遗症和多发性颅神经受累的可能性更高（*J Emerg Med*, 2013, 44: e137）。

141. 良性阵发性体位性眩晕

Benign paroxysmal positional vertigo is a common peripheral vestibular disorder. What causes BPPV?

良性阵发性体位性眩晕（BPPV）是一种常见的外周前庭功能紊乱。什么原因可以导致 BPPV？

It is caused by otoconia (small crystals of calcium carbonate), which detach from the utricular macula and fall into one of the semicircular canals. Patients have brief episodes of rotary vertigo with changes in head position.

它是由从椭圆囊斑脱离的耳石（碳酸钙小晶体）进入半规管之一造成的。患者在头部位置改变时会出现短暂旋转性眩晕（*N Engl J Med*, 2010, 362: e70）。

142. 肺支原体肺炎

M. pneumoniae is not normal pharyngeal flora, so its detection in nasopharyngeal or oropharyngeal specimens in persons with compatible illness indicates that it is the cause. What portion of community-acquired pneumonia is caused by M. pneumoniae?

肺支原体不是咽部正常菌群，所以，如果在相关患者的鼻咽或口咽样本中查到它，就可以证明它是致病原因。社区获得性肺炎中由肺支原体引起肺炎的比例是多少？

Up to 40% of community-acquired pneumonia is caused by M. pneumoniae.

高达40%的社区获得性肺炎是由肺支原体引起的(*MMWR Weekly*, 2012, 61: 834)。

143. 社区获得性肺炎应用抗生素的时间

What is the currently recommended duration of antibiotic therapy for community-acquired pneumonia?

目前建议社区获得性肺炎应该进行多长时间的抗生素治疗？

5 to 7 days. There is no evidence that prolonged courses lead to better outcomes, even in severely ill patients, unless they are immunocompromised.

5至7天。除非患者免疫功能低下，否则即使是在病情严重的情况下，也没有证据显示长期应用抗生素会产生更好的效果(*N Engl J Med*, 2014, 370: 543)。

144. 重症社区获得性肺炎最常见的致病菌

What organism is the most common cause of severe community-acquired pneumonia requiring ICU admission?

需要住进重症监护病室（ICU）的重症社区获得性肺炎最常见的致病菌是什么？

S. pneumoniae.

肺链球菌（*N Engl J Med*，2014，370：543）。

讨论：社区获得性肺炎最常见的致病菌

患者类别	致病菌
门诊治疗	肺链球菌 肺支原体 流感嗜血杆菌 肺衣原体 呼吸道病毒
住院治疗	肺链球菌 肺支原体 肺衣原体 流感嗜血杆菌 军团菌 呼吸道病毒
ICU治疗	肺链球菌 肺葡萄球菌 军团菌 革兰阴性杆菌 流感嗜血杆菌

145. 雾化治疗与血氧饱和度

Why may Sao2 fall initially during Beta-2 – agonist therapy for acute asthma?

为什么在用 β_2 受体激动药治疗哮喘急性发作时早期血氧饱和度会有所下降?

Beta-2-agonists produce both bronchodilation and vasodilation and initially may increase intrapulmonary shunting.

β_2 受体激动药可同时使支气管扩张和血管舒张，开始时可能会增加肺内分流(*Circulation*, 2010, 122: S829)。

146. 慢性阻塞性肺疾病(COPD)与预防性阿奇霉素的应用

A patient who has frequent acute COPD exacerbations despite guidelines-based treatment is a potential candidate for prophylactic use of azithromycin. Before starting prophylactic azithromycin, what testing should occur?

对即使按指南治疗还频繁发作的 COPD 患者要考虑预防性应用阿奇霉素。开始预防性应用阿奇霉素之前，应该做什么检查?

The patient should undergo electrocardiography to rule out a QTc of > 450 msec and formal audiography to exclude any hearing deficit.

患者应该做心电图检查，以排除 QT 间期 >450 毫秒的情况，还应进行正规听力检查，以排除任何听力下降(*N Engl J Med*, 2012, 367: 340)。

147. 哮喘和氦氧混合气体

Why shouldn't heliox be used for a severe asthmatic that is quite hypoxic?

为什么对于一个严重缺氧的哮喘患者不能用氦氧混合气体（Heliox）？

Because the heliox mixture requires at least 70% helium for effect, it cannot be used if the patient requires >30% oxygen.

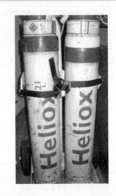

氦氧混合气（Heliox）需要至少70%的氦才能达到效果，因此它不能被用于需要 > 30% 氧气的患者（*Circulation*, 2010, 122: S829）。

讨论：医用氧

图 24　医用氦氧混合气体

按美国药典（USP）标准，医用氧（图 24）必须要用至少 99% 的纯氧气，其他为加工过程中残留的氩气和氮气。

148. 急性重症哮喘时的乳酸增高

What may explain elevated lactate levels in the setting of acute severe asthma despite the absence of infection of hypotension?

如何解释在不是因感染引起的低血压情况下，急性重症哮喘患者的乳酸水平也会升高？

Elevated lactate levels are common in the setting of acute severe asthma may be caused by excessive muscle work. Beta-agonists used in asthma treatment may also play a role owing to excessive adrenergic stimulation.

急性重症哮喘时乳酸水平升高是常见的，可能是由于肌肉过度工作所致。在治疗哮喘时用的 β 受体兴奋药可能也通过过高的肾上腺素刺激起到一定的作用（*Mayo Clin Proc*, 2013, 88: 1127）。

149. 气胸大小的定义

How does the the American College of Chest Physicians define a small versus a large pneumothorax?

美国胸科医师学会（ACCP）是如何定义气胸大小的？

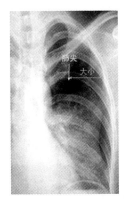

The ACCP definition of small（＜3 cm）or large（≥3 cm）PTX is based on a simple measurement of distance from the outer edge of the pleural space to the most apical portion of the collapsed lung.

美国胸科医师学会（ACCP）对气胸大（≥3 cm）小（＜3 cm）的定义是根据简单测量从胸膜外缘到萎陷肺尖部的距离来确定的，见图25（*J Emerg Med*，2013，44：457）。

图25　气胸大小的测定标志

150. 原发性自发性气胸与细针抽吸

Needle aspiration is an alternative treatment to the placement of a chest tube for patients with a first episode of primary spontaneous pneumothorax. Why should the procedure be stopped if more than 2.5 liters of air is aspirated?

作为放置胸腔引流管的一种替代手段，针穿刺抽气可以用来治疗首次发作的原发性自发性气胸患者。如果超过 2.5 L 的气体被吸出，为什么要立即停止操作？

Aspiration of more than 2.5 liters of air may indicate the presence of a persistent air leak, for which the placement of a chest tube should be considered.

抽出超过 2.5 L 的气体可能表明有持续漏气的存在，此时应考虑放置胸导管引流（*N Engl J Med*，2013，368：e2）。

151. 纵隔气肿最常见的原因

What is the most widely accepted explanation for the development of pneumomediastinum?

纵隔气肿产生的最为普遍接受的原因是什么？

Sudden rupture of distended alveoli under high-pressure gradient between the alveoli and the surrounding interstitial space; the free air then dissects from the ruptured alveoli along the bronchovascular sheaths to the mediastinum.

由于肺泡和周围间质空隙之间压力差的增加导致扩张肺泡的突然破裂，然后游离气体由破裂的肺泡，沿支气管血管鞘扩散到纵隔（*J Emerg Med*, 2013, 44：e81）。

152. 急性肺栓塞与咳血

How does acute pulmonary embolism cause hemoptysis?

急性肺栓塞如何引起咯血？

Acute pulmonary embolism can cause distention of the pulmonary vessels, leading to rupture with resulting hemoptysis.

急性肺动脉栓塞可引起肺血管扩张，破裂后导致咯血（*Mayo Clin Proc*, 2012, 87：497）。

153. 肺栓塞的胸片表现

The main value of chest X-ray in the assessment of patients with symptoms suggestive of a pulmonary embolism is to help exclude other causes of the presentation. However, there are a few signs seen that are suggestive of PE. Name them (3).

在评估有肺栓塞症状的患者时,胸部 X 线片的主要价值是帮助排除其他产生这些症状的原因。但是,也有几个征象提示肺栓塞。它们是什么(列出 3 个)?

Fleischner's sign-a prominent central pulmonary artery due to its distension by a large embolism; Westermark sign-area of oligemia distal to the embolism; Hampton's hump-a pleural-based wedge-shaped consolidation.

Fleischner 征——由于大的栓塞引起的中心肺动脉隆突;Westermark 标志——栓塞远端肺血量减少;Hampton's 驼峰征——一个以胸膜为基底的楔形实变(*J Emerg Med*, 2012, 42: 698)。

 ## 154. 汉普顿驼峰征

What is Hampton's hump? What does it signify?

什么是汉普顿驼峰征?它有什么意义?

A Hampton's hump is a peripheral wedge-shaped opacification abutting the pleura on chest x-ray, signifying pulmonary infarction distal to a pulmonary embolism.

汉普顿驼峰征是胸部 X 线片显示的一个以胸膜为基底的肺外围楔形高密度阴影,标志着肺栓塞远端肺组织已有梗死 (*N Engl J Med*, 2013, 368: 2219)。

 ## 155. 肺栓塞栓子的大小可以预测死亡风险?

Not surprisingly, hypotension due to acute pulmonary embolism predicts high early mortality. The absence of hemodynamic decompensation identifies patients who are unlikely to die from PE. How does the size of the embolus predict risk?

毫不奇怪,伴有低血压的急性肺栓塞(PE)标志着较高的早期死亡率。没有血流动力学失代偿的患者通常不太可能死于 PE。栓子的大小可以预测死亡风险吗?

The size of the emboli does not predict risk.

栓子的大小并不能预测死亡风险(*N Engl J Med*, 2014, 370: 1457)。

156. 肺栓塞溶栓并发症

According to meta-analysis of available studies on thrombolytic therapy for pulmonary embolism, what is the intracranial hemorrhage rate? What was the principal risk factor predcting for development of ICH?

根据肺栓塞溶栓治疗研究的文献分析，颅内出血发生率是什么？预测颅内出血的主要危险因素又是什么？

Meta-analysis of studies on thrombolytic therapy in PE found an ICH rate of 2%, with a mortality rate of 0.5%. Diastolic hypertension was the principal risk factor in predicting development of ICH.

肺栓塞溶栓治疗的文献分析研究表明，溶栓后脑出血率为2%，死亡率为0.5%。舒张压增高是预测颅内出血的最主要因素（*Ann Emerg Med*, 2013, 57: 646)。

 157. 急性肺栓塞与心肌肌钙蛋白

Why does cardiac troponin elevation occur in the setting of acute pulmonary embolism?

为什么急性肺栓塞会导致心肌肌钙蛋白增高？

Cardiac troponin elevation in PE is believed to result from pulmonary vascular obstruction and vasoconstriction that causes a sudden increase in pulmonary vascular resistance, pulmonary artery pressure, and RV afterload.

急性肺栓塞的心肌肌钙蛋白增高是因为肺血管阻塞和血管收缩产生的肺血管阻力，肺动脉压和右室后负荷突然升高所致(*J Am Coll Cardiol*, 2012, 60: 2427)。

158. 肺 CT 血管造影与肺栓塞预后

The information provided by CTA is not only used to confirm the presence or absence of pulmonary embolism, it can also be used for risk stratification in PE patients. What CTA findings correlate with prognosis?

CT 血管造影(CTA)所提供的信息不仅是用来确认肺栓塞的存在与否，也可以用来对 PE 患者进行危险因素分析。那么 CTA 的哪些结果与预后有关？

Some guidelines already consider CTA-documented RV dilation as a surrogate marker in risk stratification. In addition, the degree of obstruction has been shown to correlate with prognosis.

一些指南已经用 CTA 显示的右心室扩张作为危险因素的指标。此外，血栓梗死的程度已被证实与预后有关(*Exp Clin Cardiol*, 2013, 18: 129)。

159. PE 时如何应用 tPA 和肝素

You diagnose a patient in the ED with an acute pulmonary embolism and start IV unfractionated heparin. The patient then becomes hemodynamically unstable and a decision is made to administer thrombolytic therapy. What do you do with the heparin?

您在急诊科诊断一个患者患有急性肺栓塞，并开始静脉使用普通肝素。患者随后出现血液动力学不稳定，你决定进行溶栓治疗。那么你应该如何处理肝素呢？

It is recommended thatthe IV UFH is suspended during tPA infusion. Upon tPA completion, the APTT should be checked. If it is < than 80 seconds, UFH should be reinitiated as a continuous infusion without a bolus.

建议在静脉给予组织型纤溶酶原激活剂(tPA)时要暂停静脉注射普通肝素。在 tPA 治疗完成后，查激活的部分凝血活酶时间(APTT)值。如果 APTT < 80 秒，应重新开始静脉持续输注普通肝素，不需要再给负荷剂量(静脉注射量)(*Mayo Clin Proc*, 2009, 84: 11, 20)。

160. 为什么非典型肺炎的病原体被称为"非典型"?

Why are the atypical pneumonia pathogens referred to as atypical?

为什么非典型肺炎的病原体被称为"非典型"?

They are "atypical" in the sense that they are not detectable on Gram stain or cultivatable on standard bacteriologic media (Clin Inf Dis, 44: S27).

他们之所以被称为"非典型",是因为它们是无法用革兰染色检测出来或用标准细菌培养基培养出来病菌的一类肺炎(*Clin Inf Dis*, 2007, 44: S27)。

 161. 骨折后脂肪栓塞

Fat embolism syndrome occurs most commonly after long bone fracture. How long after injury does fat embolism syndrome typically manifest?

脂肪栓塞综合征最常发生在长骨骨折后。典型的脂肪栓塞综合征通常在伤后多久出现?

Fat embolism syndrome typically manifests 24 to 72 hours after the injury and rarely occurs as early as 12 hours after the inciting event.

脂肪栓塞综合征通常在伤后 24~72 小时发生,个别的也可能在外伤发生后 12 小时内出现(*Am J Emerg Med*, 2013, 31: 14, 20. e1)。

讨论:脂肪栓塞综合征经典的 3 个特征

渐进性呼吸衰竭
神经功能恶化
点状出血,皮疹

162. 手术或导管肺动脉血栓清除术

In patients with acute PE associated with hypotension, when might surgical pulmonary embolectomy or catheter-assisted thrombus removal be considered, provided such expertise and resources are available?

患者有急性肺栓塞伴有低血压，在条件和资源具备的情况下，什么时候可以考虑行肺外科手术取栓或导管介入血栓清除术？

（Ⅰ）contraindications to thrombolysis, （Ⅱ）failed thrombolysis, or （Ⅲ）shock that is likely to cause death before systemic thrombolysis can take effect（eg, within hours）.

①有溶栓禁忌证时；②溶栓失败时；③在静脉溶栓产生效果（例如在几个小时内）前可能因休克造成死亡时（*Chest*, 2012, 141（2_suppl）：7S）。

163. 胸腔积液

Overall, CHF is the most common cause of pleural effusions; it causes a transudative effusion and is most often bilateral. What is the second most common cause of a pleural effusion?

总体而言，充血性心力衰竭（CHF）是造成胸腔积液最常见的原因，它会导致漏出性积液，并常为双侧性。胸腔积液的第二个最常见的原因是什么？

Pneumonia is the second most common cause of a pleural effusion.

肺炎是第二个最常见的造成胸腔积液的原因（*Mayo Clin Proc*, 2011, 86：e10）。

164. 血培养阳性率

Blood cultures are positive in what portion of cases of severe sepsis? What about cultures from all sites?

严重脓毒症病例的血培养阳性率有多少？所有部位的培养又怎样？

Blood cultures are typically positive in only 1/3 of cases, and in up to a third of cases, cultures from all sites are negative.

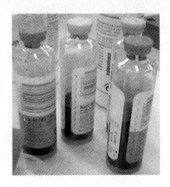

严重脓毒症通常只有 1/3 的病例血培养是阳性。有将近 1/3 的病例全部培养都是阴性(*N Engl J Med*, 2013, 369: 840)。

讨论: 如何提高血培养阳性率?

图26　血培养所获得的血标本

1. 无菌操作, 以减少污染。

2. 所有的培养都要争取在没使用抗生素前做。

3. 抽血量要足够: 成人10mL, 儿童2.5~10mL, 婴儿0.5~1mL(图26)。

4. 至少要做两套, 从不同的部位抽取血液标本。

 165. 发热性中性粒细胞减少

What is the current definition of febrile neutropenia?

发热性中性粒细胞减少目前是如何定义的?

Febrile neutropenia is defined as an absolute neutrophil count less than 500 /μL and temperature greater than 100.4℉ (38.0℃).

发热性中性粒细胞减少目前被定义为中性粒细胞绝对计数小于 500/μL 和体温高于 100.4℉（38.0℃）（*Ann Emerg Med*，2014，63：48）。

 ## 166. 化疗后发热性中性粒细胞减少出现时间

Most episodes of febrile neutropenia occur in patients receiving chemotherapy. When does the neutrophil nadir typically occur after the last dose?

发热性中性粒细胞减少大部分发生在接受化疗的患者。通常在最后一次给药后什么时间中性粒细胞最低？

For most outpatient chemotherapy, the neutrophil nadir typically occurs 5 to 10 days after the last dose.

对于大多数的门诊化疗，中性粒细胞最低点通常发生在最后一次给药后 5 ~ 10 天（*Mayo Clin Proc*，2006，81：843）。

 ## 167. 粒细胞刺激因子与发热性中性粒细胞减少症

When a patient presents to the ED with febrile neutropenia, should granulocyte colony-stimulating factor be routinely administered as part of the management?

当一个发热性中性粒细胞减少症的患者来到急诊科就诊时，粒细胞刺激因子应该作为常规治疗的一部分吗？

No. However, G-CSF should be considered in patients at high risk such as those with expected prolonged or profound neutropenia (ANC ＜100 cells/μL).

不需要。只有对高危患者才考虑用粒细胞集落刺激因子（G-CSF），如患者存在可能的长期或严重的中性粒细胞减少（ANC ＜100/μL）（*Mayo Clin Proc*，2013，88：866）。

168. 盲肠炎 (中性粒细胞减少性肠炎)

What is typhlitis?

盲肠炎是什么?

Typhlitis (neutropenic enterocolitis) is an inflammation of the bowel-usually the cecum-that occurs in the setting of neutropenia. Diagnostic criteria include the triad of fever, abdominal pain, and neutropenia.

盲肠炎(中性粒细胞减少性肠炎)是肠道炎症通常发生在盲肠段伴有中性粒细胞减少的一种疾病,其诊断标准包括三联征:发烧、腹痛、中性粒细胞减少 (*Mayo Clin Proc*, 2013, 88: 866)。

讨论:盲肠炎

机制	最常见于有中性粒细胞减少的恶性血液病患者,是由于对细胞具有毒性的化疗造成肠黏膜损伤所致
诊断	腹部 CT 是首选的诊断手段,显示扩张、增厚,并有液体潴留的盲肠
治疗	补液,抗生素,手术

169. 医院获得性和社区获得性 MRSA

How do hospital-acquired (HA-MRSA) and community-acquired (CA-MRSA) MRSA differ in terms of resistance to antibiotic classes?

医院获得性耐甲氧西林金黄色葡萄球菌(HA-MRSA)和社区获得性耐甲氧西林金黄色葡萄球菌(CA-MRSA)抗生素耐药性方面有什么不同?

HA-MRSA isolates are likely to be resistant to three or more antibiotic classes, whereas literature suggests that CA-MRSA is usually only resistant to Beta-lactams and macrolides.

HA-MRSA 菌株很可能对三类或更多类抗生素具有抵抗性,而有文献提示,

CA-MRSA 通常只对 β 内酰胺类和大环内酯类抗生素耐药（*Am J Emerg Med*，2014，32：135）。

讨论：HA-MRSA 和 CA-MRSA 的区别

医院获得性 MRSA	社区获得性 MRSA
主要发生在医院	主要发生在社区
免疫力低下或慢性病	免疫力正常
对多类抗生素具有抵抗性	只对 β 内酰胺类和大环内酯类耐药
导致所有的感染	75% 为软组织感染
与杀白细胞毒素 PVL 无关	与杀白细胞毒素 PVL 有关
严重程度各异	严重感染

 # 170. 神经氨酸酶抑制药治疗流感的好处

According to available literature, what is the benefit of neuraminidase inhibitors for acute influenza?

根据现有的文献，治疗急性流感的神经氨酸酶抑制药的好处是什么呢？

Patients who received neuraminidase inhibitors for acute influenza within 48 hours of symptom onset began to have symptom resolution approximately 1 daysooner compared with those who received placebo.

与那些接受安慰剂的患者相比，急性流感症状发作后 48 小时内接受了神经氨酸酶抑制药的患者，症状可提前 1 天缓解（*Ann Emerg Med*，2014，63：54）。

讨论：

1. 神经氨酸酶是流感病毒颗粒表面的一种由蛋白构成的酶，是病毒复制和扩散最关键的酶。

2. 神经氨酸酶抑制药（Nueraminidase inhibitor）是继金刚烷胺和流感疫苗后的一类全新作用机制的流感防治药，能选择性地抑制呼吸道病毒表面神经氨酸酶的活性，阻止子代病毒颗粒在人体细胞的复制和释放。

3. 目前神经氨酸酶抑制药有奥司米韦（Oseltamivir）和扎那米韦（Zanamivir），临床和实验室都观察到它们具有降低流感病毒感染的能力，并对 A 型、B 型流感均有疗效，且不良反应少。

171. 流感疫苗

What is the duration of immunity conferred by the influenza vaccine?

流感疫苗免疫的持续时间是多久？

Protection against viruses that are antigenically similar to those contained in the vaccine extends at least for 6 – 8 months, particularly in nonelderly populations.

防护与疫苗中的抗原相似的病毒感染的时间可延伸至 6~8 个月，特别是在非老年人群中（*MMWR Weekly*，2013，62：757）。

172. 腹泻的主要原因

What is the principal cause of gastroenteritis in the US, responsible for approximately 50% of outbreaks of diarrhea and 26% of cases of diarrhea in emergency departments?

在美国，导致50%暴发性腹泻和26%急诊科腹泻病例的主要病因是什么？

Noroviruses.

诺如病毒（*N Engl J Med*，2014，370：1532）。

173. 食源性腹泻的食物

What is the single most common food item that is responsible for diarrhea due to foodborne infection in the US?

在美国，最常见的导致食源性腹泻的食物是什么？

Contaminated leafy green vegetables are the most common single food item responsible for diarrhea due to foodborne infection (22% of cases). Noroviruses are the most common pathogens in diarrhea due to foodborne infection.

被污染的绿叶蔬菜是导致食源性腹泻的最常见食物（占22%），诺如病毒是导致食源性腹泻最常见的病原体（*N Engl J Med*, 2014, 370: 1532）。

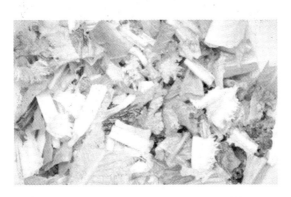

图27　各种蔬菜

 174. 容易导致难辨梭状芽胞杆菌感染的抗生素

Which antibiotics are associated with the highest risk for development of Clostridium difficile Infection?

什么抗生素最容易发生难辨梭状芽胞杆菌感染？

2 recent meta-analyses found greatest risk with clindamycin, high with fluoroquinolones & cephalosporins, moderate with sulfonamides, macrolides, & penicillins. TCN did not increase risk.

最近的两项荟萃分析发现，难辨梭状芽胞杆菌感染风险最高的是克林霉素，风险高的有喹诺酮类和头孢菌素类，中度风险为磺胺类、大环内酯类和青霉素类。四环素并没有增加难辨梭状芽胞杆菌感染的风险（*Antimic Agents Chemother*, 2013, 57: 2326）。

175. 严重难辨梭状芽胞杆菌感染的定义

Oral vancomycin or fidaxomicin are preferred for the treatment for Clostridium difficile infection in the setting of severe clinical illness. What defines severe illness?

万古霉素或非达霉素口服是治疗严重的难辨梭状芽胞杆菌感染(CDI)的首选药。严重疾病的定义是什么?

Severe CDI is defined as the presence of important comorbidity, altered sensorium, unstable clinical course, confinement in an ICU, renal failure, serum albumin < 2.5 g/dL, hypotension, or WBC > 15, 000/mm^3.

严重 CDI 的定义是有下列情况存在:重要合并症,神志改变,临床状况不稳定,住在 ICU,肾衰竭,血清白蛋白 < 2.5 g/L,低血压,或 WBC > 15 × 10^9/L(*Clin Gastroent Hepat*, 2013, 11: 1216)。

176. 感染难辨梭状芽胞杆菌后的复发率

What is the risk of recurrent Clostridium difficile infection in patients with first CDI?

患者第一次感染难辨梭状芽胞杆菌(CDI)后复发的风险是多少?

The risk of recurrent CDI is 20% to 30% in patients with first CDI and increases up to 60% after 3 or more infections.

患者第一次感染 CDI 后复发的概率为 20% ~ 30%, 3 次以上感染的复发率将增至 60%(*Mayo Clin Proc*, 2014, 89: 107)。

177. 甲硝唑治疗难辨梭状芽胞杆菌感染

Metronidazole is preferred for mild to moderate Clostridium difficile infection (CDI). The drug essentially is absorbed completely in the upper gut, resulting in very low drug levels in the colon, the major site of CDI. How, then, is it effective?

甲硝唑是轻度至中度的难辨梭状芽胞杆菌感染(CDI)治疗的首选药。药物基本上在上消化道被完全吸收,达到 CDI 主要位置结肠时的浓度会非常低。那么,它是如何发生作用的呢?

With CDI-induced diarrhea, fecal levels of metronidazole reach bactericidal concentrations against C difficile due to shorter transit time and due to diffusion of drug into the inflamed gut from systemic circulation.

CDI 引起腹泻患者大便中的甲硝唑水平能够达到杀菌浓度,是因为粪便通过时间较短和药物通过全身血液循环扩散到发炎的肠道内(*Clin Gastroent Hepat*, 2013, 11: 1216)

178. 急性艾滋病病毒(HIV)感染期的定义

The highly infectious phase of acute HIV infection contributes disproportionately to HIV transmission. How is this phase defined?

急性艾滋病病毒(HIV)感染期的传染性很强,在其传播中起到相当大的影响。这一期是怎么定义的?

The highly infectious phase of acute HIV infection is the interval between the appearance of HIV ribonucleic acid in plasma and the detection of HIV – 1-specific antibodies.

具有高度传染性的急性 HIV 感染期是血浆中出现 HIV 核糖核酸到出现 HIV – 1 特异性抗体之间的时间段(*Ann Emerg Med*, 2014, 58: 56)。

179. 艾滋病暴露前的预防

An IV drug user in the ED asks about preexposure prophylaxis for HIV prevention. Preexposure prophylaxis may be considered for adults at very high risk for HIV acquisition. According to the CDC, what places an IV drug user at very high risk for HIV?

一个静脉使用毒品者在急诊科询问有关艾滋病暴露前的预防方法。艾滋病暴露前的预防方法可考虑在感染 HIV 风险非常高的成人中应用。根据美国疾病预防与控制中心(CDC)颁布的标准,什么样的静脉使用毒品者感染艾滋病病毒的风险非常高?

Reported injection practices that place persons at very high risk for HIV acquisition include sharing of injection equipment, injecting one or more times a day, and injection of cocaine or methamphetamine.

有报告显示,增加静脉使用毒品者感染艾滋病病毒的风险包括:共享注射用品,每天注射一次或多次,以及同时注射可卡因或者甲基苯丙胺 (*MMWR Weekly*, 2013, 62: 457)。

180. HIV 血清学转化

When evaluating a patient for postexposure prohylaxis after HIV exposure, the clinician should be aware that virtually all HIV seroconversions are detectable within what time period following exposure?

当评估一个 HIV 接触后要进行预防性治疗的患者时,临床医生应该知道,在接触后什么时间内几乎所有的 HIV 血清学转化都会检测出来?

The majority of HIV seroconversions are detectable within 6 to 12 weeks, and virtually all are detectable by 6 months (NEJM, Vol. 361, 1772).

绝大部分的 HIV 血清学转化出现在6~12周内,几乎所有的都会在6个月内检测出来 (*N Engl J Med*, 2009, 361: 1772)。

181. 急性 HIV 患者应做什么检查?

A febrile illness with oral or genital ulcers is highly suggestive of acute HIV. Patients suspected of having acute HIV should have what labs obtained?

伴口腔或生殖器溃疡的发热性疾病要高度怀疑急性艾滋病病毒感染。怀疑有急性 HIV 感染的患者应该做哪些实验室检查?

Patients suspected of acute HIV should have an HIV RNA quantification and a screening HIV EIA test. In acute infection, the plasma HIV RNA level is usually more than 50,000 copies/mL and the EIA test result is negative (Mayo Clin Proc, 12/13, 1468).

对怀疑急性艾滋病病毒(HIV)感染的患者应该做艾滋病病毒脱氧核糖核酸(HIV – RNA)定量和艾滋病病毒酶联免疫吸附(HIV – EIA)筛查试验。在急性感染时,血浆 HIV – RNA 水平通常超过 50000 拷贝/mL,而 HIV – EIA 筛查试验结果为阴性(*Mayo Clin Proc*, 2013, 88: 1468)。

 182. 什么时候开始 HIV 抗病毒治疗?

You are caring for a patient in the ED who is known to be HIV positive, but is not taking any medication. Antiretroviral treatment for HIV should be initiated when the CD4 lymphocyte count reaches what threshold?

你在急诊科治疗一个 HIV 阳性但没有服用任何药物的患者。当 CD4 淋巴细胞计数达到什么水平时应该开始抗逆转录病毒治疗?

Antiretroviral treatment is now recommended for all patients with HIV regardless of their CD4 lymphocyte count to prevent both progression and spread of the disease.

目前建议对所有的 HIV 患者给予抗病毒治疗,不管他们的 CD4 淋巴细胞计数如何,以防止疾病的进展和传播(*Mayo Clin Proc*, 2013, 88: 1468)。

183. 甲型肝炎的潜伏期

Household or sexual contact with an acute hepatitis A case is the most commonly reported risk for infection. What is the incubation period for Hepatitis A?

通过家人密切接触或性接触传播的急性甲型肝炎是文献报道中最常见的感染途经。甲型肝炎潜伏期是多长？

The incubation period is 14 to 28 days (up to 50 days).

潜伏期为 14～28 天（最多 50 天）(*Clin Liver Dis*, 2013, 2: 227)。

184. 急性肝炎的转氨酶变化

With viral hepatitis, when do the AST and ALT levels peak? When do they return to normal?

患病毒性肝炎时，血清天门冬氨酸氨基转移酶（AST）和血清丙氨酸氨基转移酶（ALT）什么时候达到高峰？什么时候恢复到正常？

With viral hepatitis, AST and ALT levels increase over 1 to 2 weeks to levels in the thousands, and return to normal in 6 weeks in uncomplicated cases.

患病毒性肝炎时，AST 和 ALT 在 1～2 周后升高到数千单位水平，在没有合并症的病例中它们将在 6 周内恢复到正常(*EMCNA*, 2011, 29: 293)。

185. 活动性丙肝

A patient's HCV antibody test returns as reactive. How does one differentiate between current and past Hepatitis C infection?

一个患者的丙肝病毒抗体检查报告有异常。如何区分现在有感染还是既往有过感染？

A positive test for HCV RNA identifies current infection.

丙型肝炎病毒脱氧核糖核酸（HCV - RNA）试验阳性，说明患者现在已感染（*MMWR Weekly*, 2013, 62：362）。

186. 丁型肝炎

What is Hepatitis Delta?

什么是丁型肝炎？

Hepatitis Delta, which is caused by infection of hepatitis B surface antigen (HBsAg)-positive individuals with the hepatitis D virus (HDV), is considered the most severe form of chronic viral hepatitis.

丁型肝炎是由乙肝表面抗原（HBsAg）阳性者被丁型肝炎病毒（HDV）感染，被认为是慢性病毒性肝炎最严重的形式（*Clin Liver Dis*, 2013, 2：237）。

187. 单核细胞增多症的诊断

Heterophile IgM antibodies are measurable in 75% of patients in the 1st week of mononucleosis illness. If you have a high clinical suspicion for mononucleosis and feel it is important to establish the diagnosis, what is the next test to order?

75%的单核细胞增多症患者在第1周内可测到嗜异性凝集试验 IgM 抗体。如果你有一个患者，临床上高度怀疑为单核细胞增多症，并且需要明确诊断，下一步应做什么检查？

If the heterophile Ab is negative and there is a high suspicion for mononucleosis, order EBV-specific antibodies; EB viral IgM antibodies are diagnostic for acute infection (97% sensitivity, 94% specificity).

如果嗜异性凝集试验抗体阴性，又高度怀疑为单核细胞增多症，可查 EBV 特异性抗体；EB 病毒 IgM 抗体对急性感染有诊断价值（敏感性 97%，特异性 94%）（*Mayo Clin Proc*，2012，87：e101）。

 ## 188. EB 病毒感染患者的肝功能异常

Elevated liver enzymes occur in 80% – 90% of patients with EBV infections (e. g. infectious mononucleosis). When do they commonly peak? When do they typically normalize?

肝脏酶谱升高可以发生在 80% ~90% 的 EB 病毒感染的患者（如传染性单核细胞增多症）中。它们通常什么时候达高峰？什么时候恢复正常？

They commonly peak 2 to 3 weeks after symptom onset, and normalize within 3 to 6 weeks after symptom onset.

它们通常在症状出现后 2 ~3 周达高峰，3 ~6 周内恢复正常（*Mayo Clin Proc*，2012，87：e101）。

 ## 189. 麻疹样皮疹与单核细胞增多症

Morbilliform rashes are well described in patients with infectious mononucleosis treated with amoxicillin or ampicillin. How common is this phenomenon? Does it occur with other Beta-lactam antibiotics?

传染性单核细胞增多症患者在应用阿莫西林或氨苄西林后会出现麻疹样皮疹，这一现象已有很好的描述。这种现象常见吗？是否也可以由其他 β 内酰胺类抗生素引起？

Morbilliform rashes occur in up to 95% of mononucleosis patients treated with amoxicillin or ampicillin and in 40 – 60% of mononucleosis patients treated with other Beta-lactams.

麻疹样皮疹高达 95% 发生在经阿莫西林或氨苄西林治疗后的患者中；40% ~60% 发生于使用其他 β 内酰胺类抗生素的单核细胞增多症患者（*N Engl J Med*，2010，362：1993）。

190. 自发性细菌性腹膜炎的诊断

What cell count on peritoneal fluid analysis supports a diagnosis of spontaneous bacterial peritonitis?

腹腔液分析时多少细胞计数支持自发性细菌性腹膜炎（SBP）的诊断？

The diagnosis of SBP requires 250 or more neutrophils.

自发性细菌性腹膜炎（SBP）的诊断需要 250 以上的中性粒细胞（*Mayo Clin Proc*，2013，88：e115）。

191. 腹膜透析患者的腹膜炎诊断标准

What level of white blood cell count on examination of peritoneal fluid in a patient undergoing peritoneal dialysis who presents to the ED with abdominal pain is consistent with a diagnosis of peritonitis?

在检查一个以腹痛到急诊就诊的腹膜透析患者的腹膜透析液时，多少白细胞计数可以诊断腹膜炎？

A white-cell count of (> 100 cells per high-power field is consistent with a diagnosis of peritonitis.

每高倍视野 > 100 个白细胞计数时可以诊断腹膜炎（*N Engl J Med*，2013，368：375）。

192. 腹膜透析患者透析管出口处感染

A peritoneal dialysis patients presents with the presence of purulent drainage indicating an exit-site. Do you remove the catheter? How are antibiotics administered to treat the infection?

腹膜透析患者在透析管出口处有脓性分泌物。你要将导管拔除吗？如何给予抗生素治疗感染？

Oral antibiotic therapy is generally recommended. Initially, uncomplicated exit-site infections do not mandate catheter removal.

一般建议口服抗生素治疗。最初，单纯的透析管出口处感染不必要将导管拔除(*Perit Dial Int*, 2010, 30: 393)。

 193. 狂犬病的原因

Although a dog bite is responsible for most rabies infections in humans in the developing world, what animal is responsible for most cases of rabies in the US?

发展中国家中，被狗咬伤是造成人类狂犬病的主要原因，在美国大多数狂犬病是由什么动物引起的？

Bats. Transmission is usually through a bite, which is often unrecognized. Rabies can also be transmitted by aerosolized exposure, such as could occur in a cave with a very large density of bats.

蝙蝠。通常是由于容易被忽视的咬伤来传播。狂犬病还可以通过空气传播，如在一个蝙蝠密集的山洞里(*N Engl J Med*, 2013, 368: 172)。

 194. 狂犬病可以通过人与人传播吗？

Does human-to-human transmission of rabies occur?

狂犬病可以通过人与人传播吗？

Human-to-human transmission is well documented only in cases of organ or tissue transplantation but is considered possible through contamination of wounds or mucus membranes with saliva, tears, or neural tissue from infected patients.

狂犬病病人与人之间的传播在器官或组织移植的情况下是大有证据的，但也可能通过由被感染患者的唾液、泪液或体液组织污染的伤口或黏膜传播(*MMWR Weekly*, 2013, 62: 642)。

195. 骨髓炎与 X 线片上的"鼠咬征"

On plain x-rays, when is the "rat bite" appearance of osteomyelitis visible following onset of signs and symptoms?

在骨髓炎症状和体征出现后多久，普通 X 线片上可出现"鼠咬征"？

The "rat bite" in bone that is often seen in osteomyelitis becomes visible on plain radiography 2 to 3 weeks after the onset of symptoms and signs.

在骨髓炎 X 线平片上常见的"鼠咬征"，通常在症状和体征出现后 2~3 周内表现出来（*N Engl J Med*, 2014, 370: 353）。

196. 头孢菌素过敏的淋病患者的治疗

A 250 – mg intramuscular dose of ceftriaxone is most effective in curing gonococcal infections at both genital and extragenital sites. In patients who are allergic to cephalosporins, what is the treatment?

肌内注射头孢曲松 250 mg 是最有效的治疗生殖器和生殖器以外部位淋病奈瑟菌感染的方法。患者若是对头孢类抗生素过敏，应该如何治疗？

In patients who are allergic to cephalosporins, the only option is 2 g of azithromycin orally.

患者若是对头孢类抗生素过敏，其他的选择就只有阿奇霉素 2 g 口服（*N Engl J Med*, 2012, 366: 485）。

197. 兔热病

Tularemia is a potentially serious bacterial zoonosis that has been reported from all U. S. states except Hawaii. The etiologic agent, Francisella tularensis, is highly infectious. How is it transmitted?

兔热病是一种潜在的严重细菌性人畜共患病,据报道除了夏威夷,美国所有的州都有发生。土拉弗朗西斯菌(Francisella tularensis)病原体具有很强的传染性。它是如何传播的?

Tularemia can be transmitted through arthropod bites, direct contact with infected animal tissue, inhalation of contaminated aerosols, and ingestion of contaminated food or water.

兔热病可以通过节肢动物叮咬,接触受感染动物组织,吸入污染的空气,或食入污染的食物或水传播(*MMWR Weekly*, 2013, 62: 834)。

198. 莱姆病血清学试验

For how long can positive serologic studies persist after successful treatment in patients with Lyme disease?

莱姆病患者成功治疗后的阳性血清学试验将持续多久?

Positive serologic studies may persist for 10 – 20 years after successful treatment in patients with Lyme disease.

莱姆病患者成功治疗后的阳性血清学试验将持续 10～20 年(*Mayo Clin Proc*, 2011, 86: 245)。

199. 组织胞浆菌病

Histoplasmosis is caused by infection with the fungus, Histoplasma capsulatum, following inhalation of contaminated soil. Where is Histoplasmosis endemic in the US?

组织胞浆菌病是由人体吸入受真菌中的组织胞浆菌污染的土壤后引起的感染。组织胞浆菌病在美国哪里流行?

The recognized zone of histoplasmosis endemicity extends from the Ohio River Valley west into North Dakota and South Dakota.

公认的组织胞浆菌病流行区域从俄亥俄河谷西延伸至北达科他州和南达科他州(*MMWR Weekly*, 2013, 62: 834)。

200. 美国目前结核病的发病率

Since the resurgence of TB in the late 1980s, the US has experienced 20 consecutive years of declines in TB rates. 4 states account for half of all TB cases. Name them. In which 2 states are rates of TB the highest?

自从结核病在 20 世纪 80 年代后期再次流行后,美国已经经历了连续 20 年的结核病发病率下降。有 4 个州占所有结核病例的一半,它们的名字是什么? 哪 2 个州结核病发病率最高?

4 states (California, Texas, NY, and Florida) reported half of all TB cases in 2012. These 4 states have < 1/3 of the US population. Rates of TB were highest in Alaska and Hawaii, which combined have < 1% of the population.

在 2012 年 4 个州(加利福尼亚州,得克萨斯州,纽约州和佛罗里达州)报告了所有结核病例的一半,这 4 个州占美国人口的不到 1/3。结核病发病率最高的州是阿拉斯加和夏威夷,它们的人口还不到美国人口的 1%(*MMWR Weekly*, 2013, 62: 201)。

201. 葡萄球菌性烫伤样皮肤综合征

Why does Staphylococcal scalded skin syndrome usually occur in children?

为什么葡萄球菌性烫伤样皮肤综合征通常发生于儿童？

Staphylococcal scalded skin syndrome usually occurs in children, as adults have specific antistaphylococcal antibodies to excrete the staphylococcal toxin through adequate renal clearance.

葡萄球菌性烫伤样皮肤综合征通常发生在儿童（图28），因为成年人有特异的葡萄球菌抗体，可以通过肾脏将葡萄球菌毒素有效排除（*Mayo Clin Proc*，2009，84：838）。

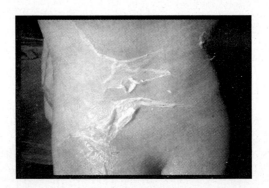

图28　葡萄球菌性烫伤样皮肤综合征的皮肤病变

202. 洛基山斑疹热的皮疹

Describe the rash of Rocky Mountain spotted fever. When in the course of the illness does it typically appear?

描述一下洛基山斑疹热的皮疹。它通常会在疾病过程中的什么时候出现？

The rash classically appears on day 2 ~ 4 of illness, first on wrist and ankles, including palms and soles, then spreading to the trunk. It is erythematous and macular in the early stages, progressing to papules and then petechiae.

洛基山斑疹热通常在病情的第 2~4 天出现，从手腕和足踝部开始，包括手掌和脚掌，然后蔓延到躯干。早期阶段皮肤发红，呈斑疹状，然后发展到丘疹和瘀斑，见图 29（*J Emerg Med*, 2013, 45：186）。

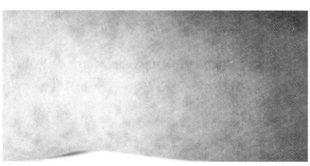

图 29　洛基山斑疹的皮肤病变

 203. 中心静脉导管感染

A patient with a central venous catheter in place presents to the ED with sepsis. Blood cultures are drawn via the catheter and from a peripheral site. How do results of blood cultures determine if the catheter is the source of infection?

一个置有中心静脉导管的患者因败血症到急诊室就诊。采集了经导管和外周静脉的血液做培养。如何用血培养的结果来确定导管是否为感染源？

In general, central venous catheters are considered infected if blood cultures drawn from those catheters become positive at least 120 minutes before peripheral blood cultures.

在一般情况下，如果来自导管的血培养比外周血培养提前至少 120 分钟呈阳性，应考虑是中心静脉导管感染（*Mayo Clin Proc*, 2013, 88：866）。

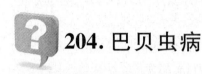

204. 巴贝虫病

A patient in whom Lyme disease has been diagnosed develops more severe disease despite treatment with standard antimicrobial therapy. What should you suspect?

一个诊断明确的莱姆病患者在标准抗菌治疗后病情出现恶化。你应该怀疑什么?

Babesiosis should be suspected in patients in whom Lyme disease or anaplasmosis has been diagnosed if more severe disease develops or if they have a poor response to standard antimicrobial therapy.

对已确诊的莱姆病或无形体病(边虫症)患者,如果出现病情加重或对标准的抗菌药物治疗反应不佳,要怀疑巴贝虫病(Babesiosis)(*N Engl J Med*, 2012, 366: 2397)。

讨论: 巴贝虫病

传播途经	由一种感染红细胞与疟原虫相似的寄生虫经蜱虫叮咬传播。
临床特点	与莱姆病相似,但对于无脾脏、老年人或免疫力低下的患者可有生命危险。
治 疗	要用抗寄生虫病药(如马拉隆)和红霉素类药物(阿奇霉素,克拉霉素)。

205. 肉毒杆菌中毒

What infection typically causes bilateral cranial nerve palsies, followed by bilateral descending flaccid paralysis over hours to days, with eventual loss of deep tendon reflexes?

什么感染通常会导致双侧颅神经麻痹,然后在数小时至数天内出现双侧下行性弛缓性瘫痪,最终导致深部肌腱反射消失?

Botulism. Foodborne botulism occurs when Clostridium botulinum spores, whichare ubiquitous, germinate and produce toxin. Germination and toxin formation require warm, anaerobic environments with low-acid, low-salt, low-sugar content.

肉毒杆菌中毒。肉毒杆菌生成孢子时将会发生食源性肉毒杆菌中毒。孢子形成的过程是不终止的，发芽并产生毒素。萌芽和毒素的形成需要温暖、厌氧及低酸、低盐、低糖的环境（*MMWR Weekly*，2013，62：529）。

讨论：肉毒杆菌中毒

分类	婴儿肉毒杆菌中毒
	食源性肉毒杆菌中毒
	伤口感染性肉毒杆菌中毒
食源性感染源	罐装不当的低酸食品:液体变混，盖变松，瓶变形或有裂痕，异味。
	没有人和人之间传播
预防	仔细检查罐装食品
	彻底烹调或加热
	做好的食物要保温(60℃)或冷藏(4℃)
症状	复视
	眼睑下垂
	呼吸或(和)吞咽困难
治疗	抗肉毒杆菌毒素
	呼吸循环支持
	对伤口感染引起的肉毒杆菌中毒彻底清创和使用青霉素

 # 206. 西尼罗河病毒(WNV)

Arthropod-borne viruses (arboviruses) are transmitted to humans primarily through the bites of infected mosquitoes and ticks. What is the leading domestically-acquired arboviral disease in the US?

节肢动物传播的病毒(虫媒病毒)，主要是通过受感染的蚊子和扁虱叮咬传染给人类。在美国国内最常见的虫媒疾病是什么？

West Nile virus (WNV) is the leading cause of domestically acquired arboviral disease in the United States.

西尼罗河病毒(WNV)是美国国内最常见的虫媒病毒病（*MMWR Weekly*，2013，62：513）。

讨论：流行性乙型脑炎(乙脑)是中国国内最常见的虫媒病毒病

简介	由与西尼罗河病毒密切相关的日本脑炎病毒感染引起,在亚洲是最常见的能够由疫苗预防的脑炎
传播途经	由感染的蚊子传播
潜伏期	5～15 天
症状	多数患者无症状,只有低于 1% 发展成临床疾病 急性脑炎是最常见的表现 神志改变,局部神经功能丧失,运动失调,癫痫,发热,头痛,呕吐
典型表现	帕金森综合征的表现,面罩样脸,颤抖,齿轮样强直,舞蹈手足徐动症
死亡率	20%～30%

207. 坏死性筋膜炎的早期临床表现

Prompt diagnosis and intervention reduces mortality and amputation rates for patients with necrotizing fasciitis, yet it is misdiagnosed initially in over half of cases. What is the most consistent feature of early NF?

及时诊断和治疗可以降低坏死性筋膜炎(NF)患者的死亡率和截肢率,早期约有一半以上的患者误诊。什么是早期 NF 最常见的特征?

The most consistent feature of early NF is that the pain is out of proportion to the swelling or erythema.

坏死性筋膜炎(NF)早期常见的表现为疼痛与红肿程度不成比例(*Br J Surgery*, 2014, 101: e119)。

 ## 208. 化脓性肌炎

What is Pyomyositis?

什么是化脓性肌炎?

Pyomyositis is a purulent infection of skeletal muscle. Staphylococcus aureus is isolated in 70% of cases. The thigh seems to be the most common location for pyomyositis.

化脓性肌炎是骨骼肌的一种化脓性感染。70% 的病例可分离出金黄色葡萄球菌。大腿似乎是出现化脓性肌炎最常见的部位 (*J Emerg Med*, 2013, 45: e79)。

讨论:化脓性肌炎

易感人群	通常发生在免疫力低下(糖尿病)和最近有病毒感染(甲型或乙型肝炎)的患者
分期	第一期为早期,主要表现为肌肉酸痛和低热 第二期为化脓期,局部出现感染性脓肿 第三期为脓毒症期,表现出脓毒症中毒症状
诊断	早期很容易漏诊(0~10天),诊断主要依靠磁共振(MRI)检查
治疗	应用抗生素(3周),有脓肿形成时要手术引流清除

 209. 闭合性腹外伤后 CT 检查

According to available literature, what portion of patients who undergo CT scanning for blunt abdominal trauma are found to have an intra-abdominal injury?

根据现有的文献,对钝性(闭合性)腹外伤进行 CT 扫描发现腹腔内损伤的比例有多少?

Only 10% – 24% of patients who have had CT scans for blunt abdominal trauma are found to have an intra-abdominal injury.

只有 10%~24% 的钝性(闭合性)腹外伤患者在 CT 扫描后发现有腹腔内损伤(*Ann Emerg Med*, 2013, 57: 387)。

 210. 腹部重点外伤超声检查

A positive FAST with free fluid suggestive of hemorrhage can be useful in determining who may benefit from exploratory laparotomy. Ultrasound can reliably detect as little as how much free fluid in Morison's pouch?

腹部重点外伤超声检查(FAST)可显示腹腔内与出血相关的游离液体,对判断患者是否应该做剖腹探查是有帮助的。在 Morrison 沟至少要有多少游离液体超声波检查方能够可靠地检测出来?

Ultrasound can reliably detect as little as 250 mL of free fluid in Morison's pouch.

在 Morrison 沟只要有 250 mL 游离液体，超声波仪就能够可靠地检测出来 （*J Emerg Med*，2013，45：402）。

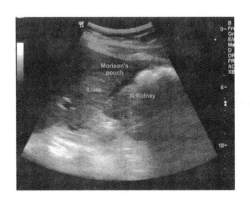

图 30　超声所测到腹腔内游离液体

 ## 211. Bryant's 体征 = 腹膜后出血

What is the significance of Bryant's sign, i. e., unilateral scrotal ecchymosis?

Bryant's 体征，即单侧阴囊淤血的意义是什么？

Bryant's sign results from blood tracking along the retroperitoneum and into the inguinal canal; it occurs in the setting of retroperitoneal bleeding and should raise concern for the possibility of a ruptured AAA.

Bryant's 体征是血液沿腹膜后进入腹股沟管所致，说明有腹膜后出血，要考虑有腹主动脉瘤（AAA）破裂（*J Emerg Med*，2011，40：e45）。

讨论：Bryant's 和 Stabler's 征

Bryant's 体征是淤血从腹股沟到阴囊，如淤血局限在腹股沟，则称为 Stabler's 体征，这两种体征都提示腹膜后出血（AAA 破裂，肝或脾破裂等）。

212. CT 膀胱造影诊断膀胱破裂

In blunt trauma cases where there is concern about a concurrent bladder injury, CT cystography is often performed after the routine CT so as to delineate bladder from arterial extravasation. How is CT cystography performed?

在怀疑有膀胱损伤和钝挫伤的情况下，为了鉴别是膀胱还是动脉漏出，通常在行普通 CT 检查后做 CT 膀胱造影。CT 膀胱造影是如何进行的？

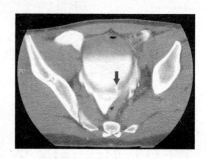

图31 CT 膀胱造影影像

CT cystography performed by first draining the bladder via the placement of a Foley catheter, filling the bladder with 350 – 400 cc of contrast material, followed by imaging the pelvis.

CT 膀胱造影是先通过放置 Foley 导尿管排空膀胱，再用 350 ~ 400 mL 造影剂充盈膀胱，然后做骨盆 CT 造影，见图 31(*J Emerg Med*, 2013, 45∶402)。

 213. 骨盆骨折的简易固定

Circumferential pelvic sheeting is a potentially lifesaving intervention for high-energy pelvic fractures that cause hemodynamic instability. The folded sheet is centered over what landmarks?

在抢救因外伤引起骨盆骨折导致血流动力学不稳定的患者时，将床单缠绕盆腔(图32)可挽救患者生命。折叠过的床单应绕过什么样的体表标记？

The folded sheet is centered over the greater trochanters, crossed anteriorly, and then pulled tightly. The ends of the sheet are secured with clamps or a knot.

折叠床单的中心应是两侧的大转子，绕过前方，然后紧紧拉住。床单的末端要用止血钳或打结固定（*N Engl J Med*，2012，369：e22）。

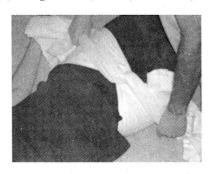

图 32　床单缠绕盆腔图像

214. 青少年运动员脑震荡

Parents of an adolescent athlete being evaluated following a concussion often ask how long the neuropsychological symptoms will last. Most with a single concussion recover to baseline within what time period?

接受脑震荡评估的青少年运动员的家长经常会问，神经心理症状将持续多久。第一次脑震荡后大多数患者在什么时间内完全恢复？

Most with a single concussion recover to baseline within 7 to 10 days and approximately 80% recover within 3 weeks.

第一次脑震荡后大多数患者在 7 至 10 天内完全恢复，约 80% 在 3 周内恢复（*JAMA*，2011，306：79）。

讨论：脑震荡后多久才能恢复运动？

1. 脑震荡症状完全消失后才能恢复运动。
2. 恢复运动的进展过程要包括循序渐进地增加与生理相适应的体育专项活动，避免直接碰撞的危险度。
3. 如随着活动的增加出现症状，要停下来，从前面没有症状的那一步重新开始。
4. 在脑震荡发生后恢复运动，一定要有经过脑震荡诊断和处理培训过的医疗服务人员的评估。

参考文献

脑震荡与体育运动：2013 年美国运动医学学会的建议. http://www. cem. org. cn/default/content/index/id/11134

第八篇　外科疾病与创伤篇

215. 脑震荡后提前恢复运动的危险

What are the short-term and long-term effects on premature return to play following a concussion?

脑震荡后恢复运动过早的短期危险和长期危险分别是什么？

The primary concern with early RTP is decreased reaction time leading to an increased risk of a repeat concussion or other injury and prolongation of symptoms.

恢复运动过早的主要顾虑是由于反应时间的减慢，会增加再出现脑震荡或其他外伤的风险，延长症状时间。另外，脑部的撞击和再次脑震荡会造成长期的神经后遗症，这是一个越来越大的顾虑（*American Medical Society for Sports Medicine*：*concussion in sports*, 2013）。

 216. 脊髓损伤

Spinal cord injury without radiologic abnormality（SCIWORA）is an injury in which the objective signs of myelopathy exist without any finding on plain films or CT scan. What is the proposed mechanism underlying SCIWORA?

没有放射学检查异常的脊髓损伤（SCIWORA）是一种只有脊髓损伤的客观体征，但在脊柱 X 线平片或 CT 扫描时没有发现任何脊髓病变的特殊情况下，SCIWORA 发生的可能机制是什么？

SCIWORA may result from self-reducing inter-segment deformity to the spinal cord or from injury to the vascular supply of the cord. It is more common in children because their bony spinal columns are more elastic.

SCIWORA 可能是由于脊髓节段间错位后自然复位或脊髓血管供应受损造成。多见于儿童，因为他们的骨性脊柱很有弹性（*J Emerg Med*, 2011, 41：252）。

217. 颈动脉夹层

New drowsiness, hemiplegia, or aphasia after concussion is a cause for concern for the possibility of a subdural or epidural hematoma. If these focal signs arenot due to intracerebral bleeding, what etiologies should be considered?

脑震荡后新出现的嗜睡、偏瘫或失语要注意硬膜下或硬膜外血肿的可能性。如果这些局部体征不是由脑出血引起的，应考虑什么原因？

A stroke from carotid artery dissection should be considered. If imaging studies of the brain and cerebral vessels show no abnormalities, a migraine-like phenomenon is presumed to be responsible for focal neurologic features.

要考虑由颈动脉夹层造成的脑卒中。如果脑和脑血管成像检查无异常，类似偏头痛的现象也可以引起局部神经功能的改变(*N Engl J Med*, 2007, 356: 166)。

218. MRI 与颈椎损伤

Recent reports suggest MRI is far superior to CT for the diagnosis of discoligamentous injury in the evaluation of cervical spine injury. What are the significant downsides to the use of MRI for the evaluation of cervical spine injury?

最近的报告表明，在诊断颈椎椎间盘和韧带损伤时，磁共振(MRI)要远远优于 CT。MRI 在评估颈椎损伤时的主要问题是什么？

Most injuries diagnosed by MRI are treated conservatively and have unclear significance; also, c-spine MRI has a false-positive rate as high as 25% – 50%, resulting in unnecessary spinal immobilization.

经 MRI 检查确诊的颈椎损伤，大多数损伤都是保守治疗，其临床意义不是很清楚。同时，颈椎 MRI 的假阳性率高达25%～50%，造成某些不必要的脊椎固定(*Ann Emerg Med*, 2012, 42: 737)。

219. Segond 骨折的临床意义

A Segond fracture is a small avulsion of the lateral tibial plateau. It has been considered pathognomic for what injury?

Segond 骨折是一种小的胫骨外侧平台撕裂伤。它一直被认为是哪种外伤的特征？

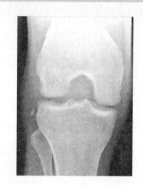

This fracture considered pathognomonic for ACL disruption. However, it should be noted that this fracture pattern is being seen with increasing frequency with PCL disruptions.

Segond 骨折被认为对前交叉韧带（ACL）断裂有特异性诊断价值（图 33）。然而，应该指出的是，这种骨折类型也越来越多地见于后交叉韧带（PCL）断裂（*EMCNA*, 2010, 28：861）。

图 33　Segond 骨折 X 线影像

220. 提睾反射消失诊断睾丸扭转

Absence of a cremasteric reflex is often used as evidence for the presence of a testicular torsion. However, the cremasteric reflex is absent in what portion of males with normal testicles?

提睾反射消失通常被用来作为睾丸扭转的证据。然而，提睾反射消失在正常睾丸的男性中出现的比例是多少？

It is well documented that the cremasteric reflex is frequently absent in up to 30% of males with normal testicles.

有证据证实，在有正常睾丸的男性中，有高达 30% 的人提睾反射消失（*Pediatr Emerg Care*, 2012, 28：80）。

221. 狗咬伤的抗生素预防

What antibiotics can be used for infection prophylaxis in high risk dog bites if the patient has a true penicillin allergy?

如果患者确实有青霉素过敏,那么何种抗生素可用于预防高风险狗咬伤的感染?

Effective alternatives include:(1)tetracycline (or doxycycline)plus metronidazole,(2)a third generation cephalosporin with anti-anerobic activity (e. g. ceftriaxone), or (3)dual therapy with clindamycin and a fluoroquinolone.

有效的替代药物包括:①四环素或强力霉素加甲硝唑;②具有抗厌氧活性第三代头孢菌素(如头孢三嗪);③克林霉素和一种喹诺酮类药物的混合治疗(*Br Med J*, 2007, 334:413)。

222. 感染后肾小球肾炎与血尿

Postinfectious glomerulonephritis is induced by infection with specific strains of group A Beta-hemolytic streptococci. Does it only occur following pharyngitis? How long after infection does the hematuria typically occur?

感染后肾小球肾炎多数是由 A 组 β 溶血性链球菌感染引起的。它是否只由咽炎引起？血尿通常在感染发生后多久出现？

Postinfectious glomerulonephritis is most commonly preceded by symptoms of either pharyngitis or impetigo, with a latent period from infection to hematuria of 10 and 21 days, respectively.

感染后肾小球肾炎最常发生在咽炎或脓疱病症状之后，从感染到血尿出现的潜伏期分别为 10 天和 21 天（*Mayo Clin Proc*，2009，84：72）。

223. 急性间质性肾炎的典型表现

What is the classic presentation of acute interstitial nephritis (AIN)?

急性间质性肾炎（AIN）的典型表现是什么？

The classic presentation of AIN includes fever, rash, arthralgias, and AKI, with laboratory evidence of peripheral blood eosinophilia, eosinophiluria, and low-grade proteinuria.

AIN 的典型表现包括发热、皮疹、关节痛和急性肾损伤（AKI），同时伴有实验室证据显示外周血嗜酸性粒细胞增多、嗜酸性粒细胞尿及少量蛋白尿（*Mayo Clin Proc*，2013，88：e93）。

224. 急性风湿热和肾功能衰竭

Acute rheumatic fever is an inflammatory condition of joints and subcutaneous tissue that also occasionally affects the heart and CNS. What is the underlying cause of ARF?

急性风湿热是关节和皮下组织的一种炎性改变，偶尔会影响到心脏和中枢神经系统。它造成急性肾功能衰竭(ARF)的根本原因是什么？

ARF is the result of an autoimmune response to infection with group Astreptococci (GAS), most commonly pharyngitis.

急性肾功能衰竭(ARF)是对 A 组链球菌(GAS)感染(最常见的是咽炎)产生自身免疫反应的结果(*J Emerg Med*, 2013, 45: e103)。

225. 晚期肾脏疾病的心肌肌钙蛋白 T

With the advent of high-sensitivity assays, how often are cardiac troponin T levels found to be significantly elevated in patients who have end-stage renal disease without cardiac symptoms?

随着高灵敏度检测的出现，在患有晚期肾脏疾病但无心脏异常表现的患者中，发现心肌肌钙蛋白 T 水平显著升高的频率是什么？

With the advent of high-sensitivity assays, cardiac troponin T levels higher than the 99th percentile are found in 100% of patients who have end-stage renal disease without cardiac symptoms.

随着高灵敏度检测的应用，晚期肾脏疾病但无心脏异常表现，患者的心肌肌钙蛋白 T 水平将100%的高于第99百分位(*Cleveland Clin J Med*, 2013, 80: 777)。

226. 0.9% 氯化钠注射液在横纹肌溶解症时的应用

Patients presenting with acute rhabdomyolysis often require in the neighborhood of 10 liters of fluid per day. Why might the administration of large amount of normal saline be counterproductive?

急性横纹肌溶解症患者通常每天需要 10 L 左右的液体。为什么应用 0.9% 氯化钠(NS)注射会适得其反？

NS can contribute to acidosis, due to the dilution of serum bicarbonate with a solution high in chloride ions, generating hyperchloremic metabolic acidosis. Acidosis exacerbates the renal injury associated with rhabdomyolysis

含氯离子高的液体会稀释血清碳酸氢盐，产生高氯性代谢性酸中毒，因此，大量应用 0.9% 氯化钠注射液可以导致酸中毒的产生。酸中毒会加重与横纹肌溶解相关的肾损伤(*N Engl J Med*, 2009, 361: 62)。

227. 折轴(Coude) 导尿管放置法

When inserting a Coude catheter into the bladder, how is the curved tip oriented?

当放置一支折轴(Coude)导尿管(图 34)进入膀胱时，弯曲尖端应朝向什么方向？

When inserting a Coude, the curved tip is pointing up, cephalad, and advanced with continuous pressure past any resistance point (typically in the region of an enlarged prostate).

当插入折轴 Coude 导尿管时，弯曲尖端应朝上，即朝患者头部的方向，并要用持续力度通过各个阻力点(阻力点通常在肥大的前列腺部位)(*J Emerg Med*, 2008, 35: 193)。

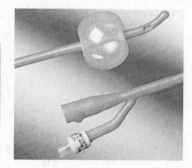

图 34　折轴(Coude) 导尿管

228. 紫色尿袋综合征

Purple urine bag syndrome presents as a dramatic discoloration of the urine bag and in patients with long-term indwelling catheters. What is its significance? How does it occur?

紫色尿袋综合征表现为长期留置导尿管的患者的尿袋出现奇迹般的变色。它的意义是什么？它是如何发生的？

The discoloration occurs in the presence of a UTI from the breakdown of tryptophan into indole by gut bacteria. Indole breakdown products interact with the plastic of the catheter bag to produce a purple coating layer.

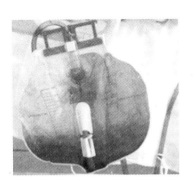

图35 塑料导尿管袋

变色的发生是由于在尿路感染时肠道细菌将色氨酸分解成吲哚所致。吲哚分解产物与塑料导尿管袋(图35)发生反应而产生紫色的覆盖层(*J Emerg Med*, 2013, 44: e335)。

229. 造影剂导致的肾病

How is contrast-induced nephropathy usually defined? What is the rate of CIN among ED patients undergoing CT angiography for pulmonary embolism?

造影剂导致的肾病(CIN)通常是如何定义的？急诊科接受 CT 血管造影诊断肺栓塞的患者中 CIN 发生率是多少？

CIN is defined as an increase in serum creatinine of 0.5 mg/dL or a relative increase of 25% above baseline several days after contrast administration. The rate of CIN is reported to be 9% – 12% in patients undergoing CTA for PE.

CIN 的定义是在给造影剂几天后血肌酐升高超过平时的 0.5 mg/L 或相对增加了 25% 以上。据报道在为诊断肺动脉栓塞而接受 CT 造影的患者中，CIN 发生率为 9% ~12% (*Acad Emerg Med*, 2013, 20: 40)。

230. 肾源性系统性纤维化

Patients with renal failure who receive gadolinium in conjunction with an MRI scan are at risk for what complication?

肾衰竭患者在接受钆增强 MRI 扫描后会有产生什么并发症的危险?

Nephrogenic systemic fibrosis, a debilitating, fibrosing disorder predominantly involving the skin.

肾源性系统性纤维化,一种主要累及皮肤的恶性纤维化病变(*Mayo Clin Proc*, 2010, 85: 1046)。

 231. 低钙血症的典型表现

What electrolyte abnormality classically causes paresthesias in a perioraldistribution?

哪种电解质紊乱会造成典型的口周麻木?

Hypocalcemia.

低钙血症(*Mayo Clin Proc*, 2011, 86: e21)。

讨论: 低钙血症的典型表现

束臂征(Trousseau's sign)
面部叩击征(Chvostek's sign)
低反射
声带痉挛
抽搐
视乳头水肿
QT 间期延长

232. Chvostek 征与低钙血症

Chvostek sign is considered to be evidence of neuromuscular hyperexcitability, and is seen as a sign of hypocalcemia. However, why is this clinical sign essentially worthless?

Chvostek 征被认为是神经肌肉兴奋性增高的表现，并且可见于低钙血症。然而，为什么这个临床体征基本上是毫无价值的？

25% of healthy individuals (43% between the ages of 20 and 29 years) have a positive Chvostek sign, and 29% of patients with hypocalcemia do not.

25% 的健康人(43% 的年龄在 20 ~ 29 岁)会有阳性 Chvostek 征，而 29% 的低钙血症患者却可能是阴性(*Neurology*, 2013, 80: 1067)。

233. 高钾和胰岛素

What is the onset of action of a single bolus of IV insulin for the treatment of hyperkalemia? When is the effect maximal?

在治疗高钾血症时，静脉注射胰岛素(一个剂量10U)的起效时间是什么？达到最大作用的时间又是什么？

An IV dose of 10 units of regular insulin to adult patients lowers the serum potassium by about 0.6mmol/L. The onset is within 15 minutes and the effect is maximal at 30 – 60 minutes.

对于一个成年患者，静脉注射普通胰岛素 10 个单位可降低血清钾 0.6 mmol/L。起效时间在 15 分钟内，大概在 30 ~ 60 分钟内达到最大效果(*Crit Care Med*, 2008, 36: 3248)。

234. 高钾和聚苯乙烯磺酸钠

When given orally for the treatment of hyperkalemia, when is the onset of action of sodium polystyrene (Kayexalate)? When does the maximum effect occur?

在口服聚苯乙烯磺酸钠(Kayexalate，降钾树脂)治疗高钾血症时，它什么时间起效？最大的效果在什么时候发生？

The onset of action is at least 2 hours and the maximum effect may not be seen for 6 hours or more.

起效时间至少要 2 小时，最大的效果可能要在 6 小时或更长时间出现 (*Crit Care Med*, 2008, 36: 3249)。

235. 肺动脉栓塞与肾病综合征

You diagnose a patient in the ED with an acute pulmonary embolism. You happen to note that the patient exhibits peripheral edema, has a low serum albumin and proteinuria. What is the diagnosis?

你在急诊科诊断一个患者为急性肺动脉栓塞。你同时也注意到，患者表现出末梢循环障碍，肢体远端浮肿，血清白蛋白低并伴有蛋白尿。你的诊断是什么？

The nephrotic syndrome is a prothrombotic condition that is a risk factor for acute PE.

肾病综合征是一种高血栓形成状态，是急性肺动脉栓塞的危险因素之一 (*N Engl J Med*, 2008, 358: 25)。

236. 如何通过腹泻的潜伏期来鉴别病毒感染和食物中毒？

In an outbreak of diarrheal illness, how does the incubation period allow you to differentiate between viral infection and food poisoning?

在腹泻爆发时,如何通过腹泻的潜伏期来鉴别病毒感染和食物中毒?

In an outbreak, the incubation period can be used to differentiate between viral infection (> 14 hours, often 24 to 48 hours) and food poisoning (2 to 7 hours).

当腹泻爆发时，可利用潜伏期的长短来区分病毒感染和食物中毒。若为病毒感染，其潜伏期一般 > 17 小时，常在 24 ~ 48 小时；若为食物中毒，则潜伏期一般为 2 ~ 7 小时 (*N Engl J Med*, 2014, 370: 1532)。

 ## 237. 上消化道出血与布拉奇福德评分

What is the significance of a Blatchford score of 0 in a patient presenting to the ED with acute upper GI bleeding?

对于一个到急诊科就诊的急性上消化道出血的患者，布拉奇福德 (Blatchford) 评分为 0 的意义是什么?

A Blatchford score of 0 effectively rules out the need for urgent intervention.

布拉奇福德 (Blatchford) 的评分为 0 可以有效地排除需要进行紧急介入检查和治疗的必要 (*Ann Emerg Med*, 2013, 62: 627)。

讨论: 消化道出血及布拉奇福德 (Blatchford) 评分

1.计分项目: 血尿素氮 (BUN)，血红蛋白，性别，心衰，肝病，晕厥，生命体征，柏油样类便
2.布拉奇福德评分分数只有为零时才有意义 (如没有突发事件并不需要介入治疗)
3.不需要放置胃管灌洗

238. 上消化道出血与黑便

Melena suggests a proximal GI bleeding source in which there is time for enzymatic breakdown to transform blood to melena. How much blood in the stomach does it take to cause melena?

黑便表明了近端胃肠道出血,因为酶有充足的时间(消化道内)将血液分解变成黑便(血红蛋白的铁氧化)。胃内需要有多少出血就会产生黑便?

In clinical experiments, placing as little as 50 mL of blood in the stomach can cause melena.

在临床实验中,仅将 50 mL 血液注入胃内便可引起黑便(*JAMA*, 2012, 307: 1072)。

讨论:上消化道出血处理要点

1. 判断上消化道出血最好的指标是肛门指检有柏油样粪便和血尿素氮与血肌酐的比值大于 30(BUV/Acr > 30)。

2. 积极治疗大出血,包括输血,早期会诊,对顽固性静脉曲张出血使用气囊压塞止血。

3. 部分少量出血的患者可以回家观察治疗,但必须要参考使用 Blanchford 的评分系统作出充分评估方能实施。

4. 有静脉曲张的患者可以放胃管,但总的来讲帮助不大。

 239. Dieulafoy 病变

A Dieulafoy lesion can cause intermittent and sometimes massive gastrointestinal bleeding. What is this lesion?

Dieulafoy 病变可导致间歇性,甚至有时为大量的胃肠道出血,这是什么病变?

Dieulafoy lesion is characterized by a dilated artery, which erodes through the gastric mucosa and bleeds. Dieulafoy lesion may occur anywhere in the GI tract but is predominantly located in the GE junction.

Dieulafoy 病变的特点是曲张动脉可通过侵蚀胃黏膜而造成出血。Dieulafoy 病变可能发生在胃肠道的任何地方,但主要位于胃与食管连接处(*Am J Emerg Med*,2013,31：889.e5)。

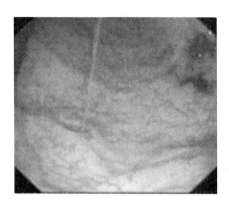

图36　**Dieulafoy** 病变

 240. 消化道出血与免疫抑制

Patients with acute GI bleeding often present to the ED. Immunosuppressed patients are at risk of acquiring opportunistic infections and several are associated with the development of GI ulcerations and GI hemorrhage. Name examples of such infections.

急性消化道出血患者经常会到急诊科就诊。如伴有免疫抑制或免疫功能低下的患者,则具有获得机会性感染的风险,其中与消化道溃疡和出血有关。举几个这些感染的例子。

Cytomegalovirus, herpes simplex virus, and fungal organisms (e. g., histoplasmosis, aspergillosis, and mucormycosis) are all associated with GI ulcerations and hemorrhage.

巨细胞病毒、单纯疱疹病毒、真菌(如组织胞浆菌病、曲霉菌病、毛霉菌病)感染都可以出现胃肠道溃疡和出血(*N Engl J Med*,2013,369：1545)。

241. 新发生腹水的鉴别诊断

The differential diagnosis for patients with new-onset ascites includes cirrhosis, CHF, and nephrosis. Approximately 10% of cases are associated with malignancy and it is most commonly associated with which cancer?

新发生腹水患者的鉴别诊断包括肝硬化、充血性心力衰竭(CHF)和肾病。约10%的病例与恶性肿瘤有关,它最常与哪种癌症有关?

Approximately 10% of cases are associated with malignancy, where it is most commonly associated with carcinoma of the ovary.

新发生腹水的患者约10%的病例与恶性肿瘤相关,最常见的是卵巢癌(*J Emerg Med*, 2012, 44: e195)。

 ## 242. 一次性抽多少腹水后要输注人血白蛋白?

Albumin infusion after large-volume paracentesis is controversial. According to current guidelines, when is albumin infusion (6 – 8 g per liter of fluid removed) recommended?

腹腔穿刺排出大量腹水后输注人血白蛋白是有争议的。根据目前的指南,什么时候输注人血白蛋白(抽出每公升液体要输6~8 g人血白蛋白)?

According to the 2012 American Association for the Study of Liver Diseases Practice Guideline, albumin infusion is recommended when more than 5 L of ascitic fluid are removed.

根据2012年美国肝病研究实践协会指南,抽出超过5 L的腹水时要输注人血白蛋白(*Hepatology*, 2013, 58: 1651)。

讨论:

腹腔穿刺排出大量腹水后输入人血白蛋白将改善腹腔穿刺后的循环紊乱、低钾,并可降低死亡率。

243. 判断胰腺炎严重程度的评分标准

How reliable are available classification systems (e. g. Ranson criteria, etc.) in predicting the severity of pancreatitis?

目前判断胰腺炎严重程度的评分标准(如 Ranson 标准等)可靠吗?

Because of the relatively low prevalence of severe disease, such clinical predictors have a low positive predictive value (43 – 49%) for the development of organ failure or serious complications.

因为严重胰腺炎的相对发病率较低,这些指标对判断发生器官衰竭或严重并发症的阳性预测值很低(43% ~49%)(*N Engl J Med*, 2014, 370: 150)。

244. 胆囊炎的超声诊断

The typical presentation of cholecystitis includes sonographic signs of cholecystitis. Name three sonographic signs of cholecystitis.

胆囊炎的典型表现包括胆囊炎的超声改变。命名胆囊炎的三种超声征象。

Sonographic evidence of cholecystitis includes gallbladder wall thickening >3 mm, pericholecystitic fluid, and sonographic Murphy's sign.

胆囊炎超声影像证据包括胆囊壁增厚 > 3 mm、胆囊周围液体及超声墨菲征阳性(*J Emerg Med*, 2014, 46: 54)。

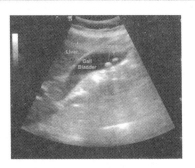

图 37　胆囊炎超声

第十篇　胃肠疾病篇

245. 如何应用乳果糖治疗肝性脑病

You intubate a patient with severe hepatic encephalopathy because he cannot protect his airway due to decreased consciousness. Lactulose is to be given via an NG tube. How often should it be given? What if NG or orogastric access is not available?

你对一个因意识丧失而不能保护呼吸道的严重肝性脑病患者进行气管插管。这时可以通过鼻饲管给乳果糖，乳果糖应该多久给一次? 但如果没有鼻胃管或口胃管时应怎么办?

Lactulose, 15 – 30 cc, can be given every 1 – 2 hours via NG tube until 3 stools are achieved. If NG or orogastric access is not available, then 300 cc of lactulose can be given in 1 L of water as an enema.

乳果糖 15～30 mL，可以通过鼻饲管每 2 小时给一次，直到患者有 3 次大便。如果没有鼻胃管或口胃管，可将 300 mL 乳果糖放在 1 L 水中灌肠（*Mayo Clin Proc*，2014，89：241）。

 ## 246. 非酒精性脂肪性肝炎与肝移植

What is predicted to become the leading cause of liver transplantation in the USA by the year, 2020? (Hint: It is not alcohol nor acetaminophen.)

在美国，到 2020 年哪种原因将成为肝移植的首要原因?（提示:不是酗酒，也不是乙酰氨基酚。）

Nonalcoholic steatohepatitis

非酒精性脂肪性肝炎（*Nature Rev Gastroenterol Hepat*，2013，10：627）。

247. 酒精性胰腺炎

For how long must a patient regularly consume alcohol before acute pancreatitis can develop?

患者必须经常饮酒多久才能造成急性胰腺炎?

The diagnosis of alcohol-induced pancreatitis (AP) should not be entertained unless a person has a history of over 5 years of heavy alcohol consumption. Clinically evident AP occurs in <5% of heavy drinkers.

除非一个人有 5 年以上的酗酒史, 否则酒精性胰腺炎(AP)的诊断不能成立。临床上明显的 AP 仅发生在 <5% 的重度饮酒者身上(*Am J Gastroenterol*, 2013, 108: 1400)。

248. 急性肾上腺危象的处理

Management of an acute adrenal crisis consists of immediate intravenous administration of how much hydrocortisone?

急性肾上腺危象的处理包括要立即静脉给予多少氢化可的松治疗？

Management of an acute adrenal crisis consists of immediate IV administration of 100 mg of hydrocortisone, followed by 100 – 200 mg every 24 hours and a continuous infusion of larger volumes of physiologic saline solution.

急性肾上腺危象的处理包括要立即静脉给予 100 mg 氢化可的松，然后是每 24 小时 100～200 mg，同时要给大量的 0.9% 氯化钠注射液静脉滴注（*N Engl J Med*, 2009, 360: 2328）。

249. 急性甲状腺功能亢进周期性麻痹

In acute thyrotoxic periodic paralysis (TPP), the most important consideration is management of hypokalemia. Although administration of IV potassium halves the duration of attack, why can this treatment be fatal in TPP?

对急性甲状腺功能亢进周期性麻痹（TPP），最重要的问题是低钾血症的管理。虽然静脉补钾可使发作持续时间减半，但为什么这种方法在治疗 TPP 时可以是致命的？

In TPP total body potassium is normal; hypokalemia results from intracellular shift of potassium. Administration of IV KCl causes rebound hyperkalemia in up to 70% of cases and consequently, fatal dysrhythmia may occur.

急性甲状腺功能亢进周期性麻痹（TPP）患者体内总的钾水平是正常的，低钾血症是由于钾向细胞内转移的结果；静脉补钾在高达 70% 的情况下导致反弹性高钾血症。因此,可能会发生致命的心律失常(*J Emerg Med*,2013,45:338)。

讨论:急性甲状腺功能亢进周期性麻痹(TPP)

1. 常见于亚洲男性,虽不常见,但却是内分泌急症之一。

2. 与低钾性周期性麻痹的临床表现相似,主要区别为甲状腺功能亢进的症状及实验室检查和家族性甲状腺功能亢进病史。

3. 在心电监护下按 0.1 g/小时静脉给予 10% 氯化钾(参与液体稀释补给),同时还须监测血清钾指标。

250. 全血细胞减少症

Pancytopenia refers to reduction in all blood cell lines. The differential diagnosis can be divided into 2 categories: intrinsic (decreased production) and extrinsic (peripheral destruction). What test in the ED can help differentiate the two?

全血细胞减少症是指所有血细胞系的数量都有减少。可分为两类：内在的（造血抑制）和外在的（外周破坏增加）。在急诊科哪些实验室检查项目可帮助区分这两大类全血细胞减少症？

A reticulocyte count-if the reticulocyte count is high, consider hemolysis or blood loss; if the reticulocyte count is low, consider deficiency in production.

网织红细胞计数——如果网织红细胞计数高，考虑溶血或失血（破坏增加，外在因素）；如果网织红细胞计数低，则考虑造血不足（内在因素）（*Mayo Clin Proc*，2012，87：799）。

 ## 251. 口服维生素 K 的指征

At what level of INR should vitamin K be administeresd to patients taking a vitamin K antagonist (e.g warfarin) if there is no bleeding?

如果服用维生素 K 拮抗药（如华法林）的患者没有出血，国际标准化比率（INR）在什么水平时应给维生素 K？

For patients taking VKAs with INRs > 10.0 and with no evidence of bleeding, it is recommended that oral vitamin K be administered.

对于服用维生素 K 拮抗药而没有出血证据的患者，当 INR 值 >10.0 时建议口服维生素 K（*Chest*，2012，141（2_suppl）：S7）。

252. 肝素诱导血小板减少症的发生时间

Heparin-induced thrombocytopenia (HIT) is a potentially life-threatening immune complication that occurs after exposure to unfractionated heparin or, less commonly, to LMWHs. Declining platelet counts begin how many days after heparin exposure?

肝素诱导的血小板减少症(HIT)是一种潜在威胁生命的免疫并发症,通常发生于使用普通肝素,少数情况下也可发生在使用低分子肝素后。血小板计数减少通常在接触肝素后几天内出现?

HIT is characterized by declining platelet counts beginning 5 to 14 days after heparin exposure.

HIT 的特点是在使用肝素后 5 至 14 天内出现血小板计数减少(*Hematology*, 2013, 2013: 668)。

253. 急性特发性血小板减少性紫癜是不可触及的

Purpura can be categorized into 2 major groups, nonpalpable and palpable. Acute ITP is characterized by the sudden onset of severe thrombocytopenia often after recovery from a viral URI. Is the purpura palpable or nonpalpable?

紫癜主要分为两种,可触及和不可触及。急性特发性血小板减少性紫癜(ITP)的特点是在病毒性上呼吸道感染 (URI)恢复后突然发生严重的血小板减少。ITP 的紫癜是可触及还是不可触及的?

Acute ITP is a common disease in children but is rare in adults. The thrombocytopenia leads to nonpalpable purpura in dependent portions of the body.

急性特发性血小板减少性紫癜(ITP)是一种常见的儿童疾病,在成人中是罕见的。血小板减少导致在下垂部位出现不可触及性紫癜(*Mayo Clin Proc*, 2007, 82: 745)。

254. 血栓性血小板减少性紫癜常见的危险因素

Thrombotic thrombocytopenic purpura (TTP) is characterized by microangiopathic hemolytic anemia and thrombocytopenia. What are the commonly described risk factors for TTP?

血栓性血小板减少性紫癜(TTP)的特征是微血管病性溶血性贫血和血小板减少。TTP常见的危险因素是什么?

Known risk factors for TTP include infection with Shiga toxin - producing Escherichia coli (STEC) and the use of drugs, including platelet aggregation inhibitors, quinine, and cocaine.

明确的血栓性血小板减少性紫癜(TTP)的危险因素包括志贺菌属毒素大肠埃希菌感染(STEC)和药物使用,包括血小板聚集抑制药,奎宁和可卡因(*MMWR Weekly*, 2013, 62: 1)。

255. 红细胞悬液的 pH

Acidosis resulting from systemic hypoperfusion exacerbates the coagulopathy associated with massive trauma. In addition, transfused blood products themselves worsen this acidosis. What is the pH of PRBCs?

外伤性全身血流灌注不足导致的酸中毒,可加重凝血功能障碍。此外,输血液制品本身也会恶化酸中毒。红细胞悬液(PRBC, 浓缩红血球)的 pH 是什么?

The pH of PRBCs decreases from 7.4 to 6.9 almost immediately after banking and falls as low as 6.7 after 3 weeks.

红细胞悬液(PRBCs)在库存后 pH 几乎会立即从7.4 降到6.9, 3 周后可低至6.7(*J Emerg Med*, 2013, 44: 829)。

256. 急性溶血性输血反应的原因

Acute hemolytic transfusion reaction (AHTR) can occur from human error resulting in mistransfusion of ABO-incompatible blood to the wrong patient. How else can it occur?

急性溶血性输血反应(AHTR)可以由于人为原因,主要发生在误输ABO血型不合血液的患者。它还能发生在其他什么情况下呢?

AHTR can also result from non-ABO antibodies in previously sensitized patients, so the occurrence of AHTR does not definitely mean human error is to blame.

急性溶血性输血反应(AHTR)也可以在以前已致敏的患者中而由非ABO血型抗体产生,所以AHTR的发生并不一定都意味着是由人为错误造成的(*J Emerg Med*, 2014, 46:341)。

257. 输血造成死亡的主要原因

What is the leading cause of transfusion-related mortality?

什么是造成与输血有关死亡的首要原因?

Transfusion-related acute lung injury (TRALI).

与输血有关的急性肺损伤(TRALI)(*Lancet*, 2013, 382:984)。

258. 输血相关急性肺损伤

Transfusion-related acute lung injury is the leading cause (approximately 50%) of transfusion-associated deaths in the US. What is the definition of TRALI?

输血相关急性肺损伤（TRALI）在美国是由输血导致死亡的首要原因（约50%）。TRALI 是如何定义的？

TRALI is defined as severe hypoxemia (room air O2 sat ＜ 90%) and bilateral pulmonary infiltrates within 6 h of transfusion initiation, with by lack of evidence of pulmonary artery hypertension or generalized fluid overload.

TRALI 被定义为在输血后 6 小时内出现严重的低氧血症（室内空气氧气饱和度＜90%）和双侧肺浸润，而又没有肺动脉高压或总体液量超负荷的证据（*J Emerg Med*, 2014, 46: 341）。

 ## 259. 上腔静脉综合征

A patient arrives to the Emergency Department with superior vena cava syndrome. No neurological symptoms are present. What is your ED treatment?

一个患者因上腔静脉综合征（SVCS）到急诊科就诊，没有神经系统症状。你应如何进行急诊治疗？

SVCS is not a true medical emergency unless neurological symptoms are present. Stenting of the SVC is effective in relieving symptoms. Chemotherapy and steroids can be used in tumors that are sensitive.

如没有神经症状，SVCS 并不是一个真正的内科急症。放置支架可以有效缓解 SVCS 的症状。化疗和类固醇可以用于对其敏感的肿瘤（*Mayo Clin Proc*, 2006, 81: 845）。

 ## 260. 弥散性血管内凝血与血小板减少

What is the significance of the finding of thrombocytopenia in a patient with severe sepsis?

严重脓毒症患者出现血小板减少的意义是什么？

Thrombocytopenia, which frequently heralds the onset of disseminated intravascular coagulation, is an independent predictor of multiple organ failure and poor outcome.

血小板减少通常发生在弥散性血管内凝血（DIC）之前，是一个独立的预测多器官功能衰竭及不良预后的指标（*Ann Emerg Med*，2006，48：54）。

 261. 溶血性尿毒综合征的发生机制

What bacterial enteric infection causes hemolytic-uremic syndrome? What is the mechanism?

什么是细菌性肠道感染导致的溶血性尿毒综合征？机制是什么？

This syndrome is caused by Shiga toxin-producing E. coli. Shiga toxin is absorbed, causing injury to endothelial cells of the glomerular capillaries with intravascular coagulation.

溶血性尿毒综合征是由产志贺菌属毒素的大肠埃希菌引起。志贺菌属毒素被吸收，损害肾小球毛细血管内皮细胞，进而造成血管内凝血（*N Engl J Med*，2009，361：1560）。

 262. 溶血性尿毒综合征最常见的原因

What is the most common cause of hemolytic uremic syndrome, which consists of hemolytic anemia, low platelets, and renal impairment?

包括溶血性贫血、血小板减少、肾功能不全的溶血性尿毒综合征最常见的原因是什么？

Exposure to Shiga toxin produced by Escherichia coli O157：H7 or Shigella species.

接触产生志贺毒素的大肠埃希菌 O157：H7 或志贺菌属（*J Emerg Med*，2012，43：538）。

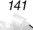

263. 凝血因子 V Leiden

What is the most common genetic risk factor for venous thromboembolism?

静脉血栓栓塞最常见的遗传危险因素是什么?

Factor V Leiden, which is present in 20% of patients with a first-time thromboembolic event. A mutation in the factor V gene results in resistance to degradation by activated protein C and leads to thrombosis.

凝血因子 V Leiden, 20%存在于首次发生栓塞的患者中。凝血因子 V 基因突变导致对活性蛋白 C 降解产生阻力, 因而促使血栓形成 (*Mayo Clin Proc*, 2011, 86: 801)。

264. 获得性血友病

It is possible to have an acquired hemophilia. How does it happen?

患获得性血友病是可能的。那么它是如何发生的呢?

Acquired hemophilia is an autoimmune disorder that often presents with severe bleeding; it results from autoantibodies against clotting factors, most often factor VIII, but antibodies against factor IX, XI, and XII are described.

获得性血友病是一种自身免疫性疾病, 常表现为严重出血。它是由抗凝血因子抗体造成, 最常见的为第Ⅷ因子, 但也有对抗凝血因子Ⅸ、Ⅺ和Ⅻ抗体缺乏的报道(*J Emerg Med*, 2013, 45: e1)。

265. 血管紧张素转换酶抑制药(ACEI)所致血管性水肿的出现时间

Is angiotensin-converting enzyme inhibitor angioedema dose dependent? Is it found almost exclusively in patients who have just started such medication?

ACEI 引起的血管性水肿与剂量有关吗？它是几乎只在刚开始用这种药物的患者中发生吗？

ACEI angioedema is a class effect and is not dose dependent, thus, symptoms can occur any time after the initial dose; up to 40% of patients with ACEI angioedema present months to years after their initial dose.

ACEI 所致的血管性水肿与药物种类相关，并不依赖剂量的大小，因此，症状可在初始剂量后任何时候发生；高达40%患者的血管性水肿发生在开始使用血管紧张素转换酶抑制药几个月到几年后(*J Emerg Med*, 2013, 45: 775)。

266. ACEI 所致血管性水肿的持续时间

For how long doesangiotensin-converting-enzyme inhibitor (ACEI) angioedema typically last?

ACEI 导致的血管神经性水肿通常持续多久？

ACEI angioedema can occur any time from a few hours up to 10 years after the initial dose; up to 40% of patients present months to years after their initial dose. ACEI angioedema typically lasts 24 – 48 hrs.

ACEI 血管神经性水肿可发生在初始剂量后任何时间，从几个小时后长达10年，通常持续24~48小时(*J Emerg Med*, 2013, 45: 789)。

讨论：

机制	血管性水肿是由缓激肽的升高造成的。
	缓激肽在正常情况下通过血管紧张素 I 转化酶和其他几种酶(如氨基酸肽酶 – P)代谢。
	氨基酸肽酶缺乏很可能导致 ACEI 性血管性水肿。
治疗	停止 ACEI 的继续使用
	H1 和 H2 拮抗药
	类固醇激素(疗效级别都不定)
	静脉应用新鲜冻干血浆(fresh frozen plasma, FFP)10 ~ 15 mL/kg;非标记使用艾替班特(Icatibant,两个都是二类推荐药);艾替班特抑制缓激肽 β_2 受体,是在结构上与缓激肽相似的 10 肽,在 ACEI 导致的血管性水肿中的效果已有个例和系列病例报道。现在正有一个前瞻性的、双盲随机、对照剂控制的临床试验在进行中。

参考文献

Wilerson G. Angioedema in the Emergency Department:An evidence-based review. Emergency Medicine Practice,Nov 2012.

 267. 急性痛风性关节炎发作

A patient presents to the ED with an attack of acute gouty arthritis? Do you stop or adjust the patient's current urate lowering therapy?

患者因急性痛风性关节炎发作到急诊科就诊,你是停止患者原治疗用药还是调整目前患者降尿酸的治疗药物?

Do not stop the patient's urate lowering therapy during an acute attack-symptoms would only worsen if it is stopped or adjusted during the flare.

急性发作期间不要停止患者原降尿酸治疗药物。如果在急性发作期间停止或调整,症状只会恶化(*Curr Opin Rheumatol*, 2013, 25:304)。

268. 超敏反应与免疫机制

If an apparent allergic reaction occurs on primary exposure to a drug, does this rule out that an immune mechanism is the cause of hypersensitivity?

如果过敏反应发生在第一次药物接触后，这是否能排除免疫机制造成超敏的原因？

No, previous contact with the causative drug is not obligatory. An immune mechanism should be considered as the cause of hypersensitivity, even in reactions that occur on primary exposure.

不能。对致敏药物的预先接触是不必须的。在考虑超敏的原因时，应该想到免疫机制，即使是在第一次接触后发生的反应(*Mayo Clin Proc*, 2009, 84: 268)。

269. 昆虫蜇伤后发生严重反应的 5 个危险因素

Name 5 factors associated with an increased risk of severe reaction from a hymenoptera sting.

说出被膜翅目昆虫蜇伤后将会发生严重反应的 5 个危险因素。

Being stung by a honeybee, underlying mast-cell disorder, a previous severe reaction, preexisting cardiovascular disease, and concomitant treatment with a beta-blocker or ACEI.

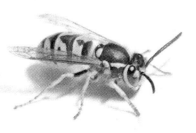

图 38　蜜蜂

被膜翅目昆虫蜇伤(如蜜蜂，图 38)的 5 个危险因素：①肥大细胞功能紊乱；②既往有严重过敏反应史；③预先存在心血管疾病；④同时服用 β 受体阻滞药或血管紧张素转换酶抑制药(*N Engl J Med*, 2014, 370:

1432）。

270. 肾上腺素的肌内注射部位

A patient presents to the ED with an anaphylactic reaction manifested by angioedema and wheezing. You determine that IV epinephrine is not indicated. How should epinephrine be administered in such a patient?

一个急诊患者因过敏性反应而出现血管神经性水肿和喘鸣。你已决定不用静脉注射肾上腺素。那么应该如何给这位患者肾上腺素呢？

Intramuscular injection in the lateral aspect of the thigh is the preferred site for administration of the drug because it is associated with more rapid absorption and increased plasma levels compared to SQ injection (Mayo Clin Proc, 8/15, e79).

大腿外侧肌内注射肾上腺素是首选部位，因为与皮下注射相比，肌内注射的吸收会更快，其血浆水平会更高（*Mayo Clin Proc*, 2013, 88: e79）。

271. 肾上腺素自动注射器注射到手指

A patient presents to the ED after self-injection of EpiPen into the finger; there is no evidence of poor digital perfusion (e. g. pain, pallor, paresthesia, prolonged capillary refill, cool temperature). What is the appropriate management?

一个被肾上腺素自动注射器（图39）注射到手指的患者来急诊科就诊，手指没有出现循环不良的证据（如疼痛，苍白，感觉异常，毛细血管再充盈时间延长，发冷）。你应如何妥善处理？

If there is no evidence of poor digital perfusion, the patient does not require any further treatment and may be discharged.

如果手指没有出现循环不良的证据，病人并不需要任何进一步的治疗，可出院观察（*Ann Emerg Med*, 2010, 56: 275）。

讨论：被肾上腺素自动注射器注射到手指的急诊处理

1. 如患者出现上述的任何缺血症状，可考虑热敷，局部用硝酸甘油膏，或局部注射 1.5 mg 酚妥拉明和 2% 利多卡因 1 mL。酚妥拉明是一个短效的 α 受体阻滞药，可以有效拮抗由肾上腺素产生的 α 受体介导的血管收缩作用。

2. 在美国无论什么时间，无论你在哪里，只要拨打 1 - 800 - 222 - 1222 就可以咨询你所在地区的中毒控制中心。

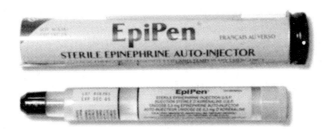

图 39　肾上腺素自动注射器

参考文献

Velissariou I, Cottrell S, Berry K, Wilson B: Management of adrenaline (epinephrine) induced digital ischaemia in children after accidental injection from an EpiPen. Emerg Med J 2004, 21:387 - 388.

第十三篇　免疫性疾病篇

272. 婴儿的明显威胁生命事件

No specific diagnosis is found at ED evaluation in 30% of patients presenting with an apparent life-threatening event. What portion of infants admitted for an ALTE need a significant intervention during hospitalization?

急诊科 30%具有生命威胁的患者没有明确的诊断。有多少比例因明显威胁生命事件(ALTE)住院的婴儿需要积极的处理?

3 recent studies have found that only 7% – 16% of infants admitted for apparent life-threatening events needed a significant intervention during hospitalization.

3 个最近的研究发现,只有 7% ~ 16% 因明显威胁生命事件入院的婴幼儿在住院期间需要积极治疗(*Ann Emerg Med*, 2013, 61:379)。

讨论:明显的危及生命的事件(ALTE)

定义	对旁观者来说是一个可怕的现象,婴儿出现呼吸暂停,皮肤颜色变化(发绀,面色苍白,红斑或淤血)、肌张力减低,哽咽或呕吐。
发生频率	大约在 1000 个新生儿中有 0.6 个。

273. 新生儿黄疸

When does physiologic jaundice in healthy newborns typically occur and when does it typically resolve spontaneously?

健康新生儿生理性黄疸一般发生在什么时候,它通常会在什么时候自动消失?

Jaundice appearing during the second to third day of life is most likely physiologic and will dissipate by the fifth or sixth day.

在出生后第二天到第三天出现的黄疸基本上都是生理性的，通常到第五天或第六天消失（*EMCNA*，2007，25：1117）。

274. 转复儿童室上性心动过速的能量

What is the energy dose for cardioversion of SVT in children?

转复儿童室上性心动过速（SVT）的能量是多少？

For cardioversion of SVT in children, use an initial dose of 0.5 to 1 J/kg. If unsuccessful, increase the dose up to 2 J/kg.

转复儿童室上性心动过速（SVT）的起始剂量为0.5～1 J/kg。如果不成功，可加大剂量到2 J/kg（*Circulation*，2010，122：S876）。

275. 小儿糖尿病酮症酸中毒时脑水肿的表现

You are caring of a young child in the ED with DKA. The patient begins to develop recurrent vomiting along with a sustained unexpected lowering of heart rate. What is your immediate concern?

你在急诊科抢救一个小儿糖尿病酮症酸中毒（DKA）患者。患者开始出现反复呕吐伴随着持续的不明原因的心率降低。你要马上考虑到什么？

In the setting of pediatric DKA, early signs of cerebral edema include headache, recurrent vomiting, and lethargy. Sustained unexpected lowering of heart rate should immediately raise suspicion for cerebral edema.

小儿患有糖尿病酮症酸中毒，脑水肿的早期症状包括头痛、反复呕吐和嗜睡。不明原因的心率降低，应立即怀疑脑水肿（*J Emerg Med*，2014，46：189）。

276. 小儿糖尿病酮症酸中毒时脑水肿的出现时间

Cerebral edema associated with DKA is rarely seen beyond the pediatric age group. When does cerebral edema typically present?

脑水肿在儿童期年龄段的糖尿病酮症酸中毒患者中很少见。脑水肿通常在什么时候出现?

Cerebral edema typically presents 4 – 12 h after initiation of therapy.

脑水肿通常在开始治疗后 4 ~ 12 小时内出现(*J Emerg Med*, 2014, 46: 189)。

277. 小儿糖尿病酮症酸中毒时脑水肿的治疗

You are managing a case of pediatric DKA in the ED. The child develops lethargy and some confusion and you are concerned about the development of cerebral edema. Do you obtain a CT scan before initiating osmotic therapy with mannitol?

你在急诊科处理一个儿童糖尿病酮症酸中毒的患儿。患儿出现嗜睡和神志模糊,你考虑可能有脑水肿,你要等脑 CT 扫描后才开始应用甘露醇渗透疗法吗?

The diagnosis of cerebral edema in the setting of pediatric DKA is mainly clinical, as initial imaging studies can be normal in 40% of patients. Initiation of treatment should precede imaging studies.

小儿糖尿病酮症酸中毒情况下脑水肿的诊断主要是靠临床表现,由于早期影像学检查在 40% 的患者中可能是正常的,因此要在影像学检查前就开始治疗(*J Emerg Med*, 2014, 46: 189)。

讨论:小儿糖尿病酮症酸中毒导致的脑水肿

死亡率	小儿 DKA 总死亡率为 0.15% ~0.51% ，但如患儿出现脑水肿，死亡率则上升到 20% ~90% 。
机制	缺血/细胞毒性 血管毒性 渗透压性(过度液体复苏的结果)
治疗	减低输液速度 甘露醇(0.25 ~1.0 g/kg，可在 2 小时内重复应用) 3% 氯化钠注射液(30 分钟内 5 ~10 mL/kg) 如运用呼吸机进行辅助呼吸，不要过度通气

278. 儿童脑膜炎球菌感染的早期表现特征

True or False: Isolated limb pain is an early presenting feature in up to 50% of children with meningococcal disease?

正确或错误:单独的肢体疼痛是儿童脑膜炎球菌感染高达 50% 的早期表现特征?

True. Isolated severe limb pain in the absence of any other physical signs in the limb is a well-established phenomenon in meningococcal disease.

正确。在没有任何其他肢体体征时，严重的肢体疼痛是公认的脑膜炎球菌感染的表现(*Emerg Med J*，2009，26：229)。

279. 新生儿正常脑脊液的白细胞计数

What is the normal CSF WBC count for a term newborn? A 4 - week old? An 8 - week old?

一个足月新生儿的正常脑脊液白细胞计数是多少? 4 周龄呢? 8 周龄呢?

The normal range for CSF WBC count are as follows: Term newborn, 0 - 22.0 - 4 weeks, 0 - 35. 4 - 8 weeks, 0 - 25.

脑脊液白细胞计数的正常范围如下：足月产新生儿$(0 \sim 22) \times 10^9/L$；$0 \sim 4$周新生儿、婴儿$(0 \sim 35) \times 10^9/L$；$4 \sim 8$周婴儿为$(0 \sim 25) \times 10^9/L$（*J Emerg Med*，2014，46：141）。

 280. 苯二氮卓类药物对小儿癫痫持续状态的治疗效果

How effective are benzodiazepines for the termination of pediatric status epilepticus (SE)? That is, in what percent of patients will cessation of status epilepticus occur for 10 minutes without recurrence within 30 minutes?

苯二氮卓类药物对终止小儿癫痫持续状态的治疗效果如何？也就是说，有多少比例的患者会在癫痫持续状态发生后10分钟停止并在30分钟内无反复？

In a just-released study of 273 patients who received either 0.2 mg/kg of diazepam or 0.1 mg/kg of lorazepam IV, with half this dose repeated at 5 minutes if necessary, 72% of cases of pediatric SE were terminated.

刚刚发表的一个研究显示，针对273例癫痫持续状态的儿童患者，在得到静脉0.2 mg/kg的地西泮或0.1 mg/kg的劳拉西泮后（如有必要，可在5分钟内重复半量），73%的儿童患者的癫痫持续状态得以终止（*JAMA*，2014，311：1652）。

 281. 儿童急性骨髓炎

Which bone is most commonly affected in acute osteomyelitis in children?

儿童急性骨髓炎最容易发生在哪块骨头？

The femur, accounting for 23 – 29% of cases. The tibia is the second most common location.

股骨，占所有病例的23%～29%。胫骨是第二个最常见的部位（*N Engl J Med*，2014，370：353）。

282. D – 二聚体在儿科中的应用

Why is use of a D-dimer level less useful in children to evaluate for acute pulmonary embolism?

为什么 D – 二聚体在评估儿童急性肺栓塞时的作用不大？

The D-dimer level is less useful in children given that the majority of pediatric patients with pulmonary embolism have underlying clinical conditions that may themselves elevate its level.

D – 二聚体在评估儿童急性肺栓塞中的作用不大，是因为多数患肺动脉栓塞的儿童都可能有使 D – 二聚体水平升高的基础疾病（*J Emerg Med*，2012，42：108）。

 283. 如何取新生儿血样

The American Academy of Pediatrics has made recommendations to reduce pain associated with ED procedures in neonates. When obtainnig blood for diagnostic testing, is heel stick or venipuncture less painful?

美国小儿科学会已经提出建议，要减少新生儿由急诊操作带来的疼痛。在采血做诊断性检查时，足跟采血（图 40）与静脉取血哪种痛苦少一些？

Venipuncture seems to be less painful than heel lancing for obtaining blood for diagnostic testing.

在采血做诊断性检查时，从静脉取血似乎比足跟采血痛苦少一些（*Pediatrics*，2004，114：1351）。

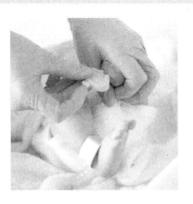

图 40　新生儿足跟采血

284. 吮吸蔗糖可减少新生儿对疼痛刺激的反应

Sucrose has been found to decrease the response to noxious stimuli such as heel sticks and injections in neonates. At what age is the use of sucrose most effective? At what age is this effect no longer effective?

蔗糖(放在婴儿奶嘴上吮吸)已被发现可以减少新生儿对于足跟取血和注射造成的疼痛反应。在什么年龄应用蔗糖是最有效的？在什么年龄用这个方法不再有效？

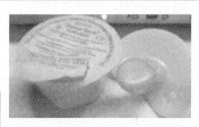

图 41 蔗糖

This effect of sucrose seems to be strongest in the newborn infant and decreases gradually over the first 6 months of life.

蔗糖的这种减少疼痛的效应似乎是对新生儿期最强，对 6 个月龄后的婴儿效果逐渐减弱(*Pediatrics*, 2004, 114: 1348)。

285. 小儿颈椎假性错位

At what age does pseudosubluxation of the cervical spine resolve?

颈椎假性错位在什么年龄消失？

8 years of age.

8 岁以下(*Ann Emerg Med*, 2012, 58: 252)。

286. 小儿第 2 颈椎齿状突假性骨折

The body of C2 fuses with the odontoid between 3 and 6 years of age, and this fusion produces a synchondrosis that appears similar to a fracture on X-ray until what age?

第 2 颈椎体(C2)和齿状突的融合在 3 到 6 岁之间开始，一直到什么年龄之前此融合产生的 C2 齿状突软骨联合在 X 线上会类似于骨折影像？

The synchondrosis is visible until 11 years of age.

第 2 颈椎体(C2)软骨联合一直到 11 岁在 X 线片上都是可见的(*J Emerg Med*, 2011, 41: 252)。

287. 手足口病的病原体

What is the etiologic agent that causes herpangina, acute hemorrhagic conjunctivitis, and hand, foot, and mouth disease?

引起疱疹性咽峡炎，急性出血性结膜炎，手足口病的病原体是什么？

Coxsackie virus.

柯萨奇病毒(*Nelson Textbook of Pediatrics*, 19th edition)。

288. 水痘的治疗

For otherwise healthy persons aged > 12 years who develop varicella, what treatment-if any-is recommended?

年龄大于 12 岁的健康人患水痘，如需要治疗的话，你有什么建议？

For otherwise healthy persons aged > 12 years who develop varicella, oral acyclovir is recommended. Treatment should be initiated as soon as possible, ideally within the first 24 hours.

年龄大于 12 岁的健康人患水痘, 建议口服阿昔洛韦。治疗应尽早开始, 最好在 24 小时内 (*MMWR Weekly*, 2013, 62: 261)。

 ## 289. 婴幼儿肉毒杆菌中毒

Infantile botulism results from ingestion of Clostridium botulinum spores; 90% of cases occur in infants < 6 months old. Infants present with vague symptoms (e. g. hypotonia, poor feeding). How often does respiratory failure occur?

婴幼儿肉毒杆菌感染是由摄入肉毒杆菌孢子引起的;90% 的病例发生在 < 6 个月的婴儿。婴幼儿的表现为非特异的症状(如肌张力低下, 厌食)。呼吸衰竭的发生频率如何?

Approximately half of all infants with infantile botulism require mechanical ventilation at some point during the course of the infection.

大约有一半的肉毒杆菌中毒的婴儿在感染的某个阶段需要机械通气辅助呼吸 (*J Emerg Med*, 2013, 45: 842)。

 ## 290. 百日咳疫苗

Childhood vaccination for Bordetella pertussis typically confers immunity for how long?

儿童百日咳疫苗接种免疫力通常会维持多久?

Immunity rarely lasts more than 12 years.

免疫力很少保持超过 12 年(*JAMA*, 2010, 304: 890)。

291. 围绝经期后状态与急性冠状动脉综合征

Why is the post-menopausal state a risk factor for acute coronary syndrome?

为什么围绝经期后状态是发生急性冠状动脉综合征的危险因素？

There are multiple reasons: rising LDL and declining HDL, rapid rise in stiffness of arteries, and decreased estrogen; estrogen helps maintain normal functioning of the endothelial layer of the vasculature.

有多种原因：低密度脂蛋白升高和高密度脂蛋白下降，动脉硬化速度加快，雌激素减少（雌激素有助于维持血管内皮细胞层的功能）（*J Emerg Med*, 2012, 43: 815）。

292. 怀孕期间脑利钠肽水平

Brain natriuretic peptide levels double during pregnancy, in part because of the increased blood volume. A value less than what level, then, should be considered normal?

在怀孕期间脑利钠肽（BNP）水平会增加一倍，部分原因是由于血容量增加。低于什么水平应该认为是正常的？

Although the BNP level doubles during pregnancy, a normal value should still be less than 100 pg/mL.

尽管脑利钠肽水平在怀孕期间增加一倍，正常值仍然应该小于 100 pg/mL（*EMCNA*, 2012, 30: 949）。

293. 围产期心肌病

What is the etiology of peripartum cardiomyopathy(PPCM)?

围产期心肌病的病因是什么？

The etiology is unknown; multiple etiologies have been proposed. The most substantiated etiology is viral myocarditis. It is thought that the relative immunosuppression of pregnancy may increase the risk of viral myocarditis.

围产期心肌病虽然病因不是很清楚，但已经提出多种可能的因素。最主要的病因是病毒性心肌炎。公认的理由为怀孕引起的相对免疫抑制增加了患病毒性心肌炎的可能性（*J Emerg Med*，2009，36：141）。

294. 孕妇与血栓形成

Pregnant women are at increased risk for thrombotic events, including deep venous thrombosis. The risk continues after delivery and has been thought to be highest during the first 6 weeks postpartum. When does it return to baseline?

孕妇是发生血栓形成的高危人群，包括深静脉血栓。其风险在分娩后还是存在的，产后 6 周内达高峰。什么时候会回到基线？

In a recent analysis of a large database of 1.7 million pregnant women, the thrombotic risk remained elevated through 12 weeks postpartum, after which time the risk was no longer significantly elevated.

最近的一个有 170 万孕妇参加的大样本分析显示，血栓形成的风险一直持续到产后 12 周，之后就不再有明显升高（*N Engl J Med*，2014，370：1307）。

295. 妊娠期静脉血栓栓塞症的抗凝治疗

Why is treatment with oral anticoagulation for venous thromboembolism (VTE) generally avoided during pregnancy?

为什么怀孕期间尽量避免用口服抗凝药治疗静脉血栓栓塞症(VTE)?

The treatment of VTE with oral anticoagulation is generally avoided during pregnancy due to the teratogenic effects in the first trimester and the risks of fetal intracranial bleeding in the third trimester.

怀孕期间尽量避免用口服抗凝药治疗静脉血栓栓塞症(VTE),因为它有致畸作用,妊娠晚期可以导致胎儿颅内出血(*Hematology*,2013,2013:457)。

 ## 296. 妊娠与主动脉夹层

When aortic dissection occurs in women < 40 years of age, about 50% are seen during pregnancy. Why is pregnancy a risk factor of acute aortic dissection?

当主动脉夹层发生在小于 40 岁的女性时,约 50% 发生在怀孕期间。为什么妊娠成为急性主动脉夹层的一个危险因素?

The increased risk is thought due to increased circulatory volume and systemic BP during late pregnancy, and a failure in collagen and elastin deposition in the aorta from elevated levels of estrogen and progesterone in pregnancy.

危险因素的增加是由于下列原因:妊娠后期循环血量的增加及全身血压的增高,加上怀孕期间由于雌激素及孕酮水平的增加使胶原蛋白和弹性蛋白不能在主动脉沉积(*J Emerg Med*,2014,46:e13)。

297.妊娠期检测母体 Rh 血型的重要性

When Rh-positive fetal blood enters the circulation of an Rh-negative mother, maternal anti-D antibodies are produced. What effects does this process, called sensitization or alloimmunization, have on the pregnancy during which it occurs?

当 Rh 血型阳性胎儿血进入一个 Rh 血型阴性母亲的血液循环时,母亲将产生抗 D 抗体。这个被称为致敏或同种免疫过程。对发生这一反应的妊娠有什么影响?

Sensitization usually has no adverse effects during the pregnancy in which it occurs but results in an amplified immune response if further maternal exposure to the D antigen occurs during a subsequent pregnancy.

致敏通常对发生致敏过程的怀孕没有不良影响,但在下次妊娠时如果再次接触 D 抗原,将产生增强的免疫反应(*Ann Emerg Med*,2013,59:285)。

讨论:

在以后的妊娠中,母体内的抗 D 抗体将进入胎儿,导致胎儿溶血(新生儿 Rh 血型溶血病)。

 298.流产后绒毛膜促性腺激素持续升高

After uterine evacuation in the setting of a miscarriage, what is the significance of a postoperative plateau or increase in serum hCG?

在行流产清宫术后,血清绒毛膜促性腺激素(HCG)水平持续或升高的意义是什么?

After uterine evacuation, a postoperative plateau or increase in serum hCG strongly suggests an ectopic pregnancy.

清宫术后血清 HCG 水平持续或升高强烈提示宫外孕(*N Engl J Med*,2009,361:379)。

299. 怀孕多久 B 超可视胎囊？

At what gestational age is a gestational sac first visible on transvaginal ultrasonography?

经阴道超声最早可以在怀孕多久时间内看到胎囊？

The gestational sac is first seen at approximately 5 weeks of gestational age, appearing as a small cystic-fluid collection with rounded edges and no visible contents.

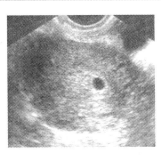

图42　B 型超声显示胎囊

大约在 5 周胎龄的时候可以看到胎囊（图 42），表现为一个球形没有内涵物的小囊性液体（*N Engl J Med*, 2013, 369：1443）。

300. 肩位难产

Shoulder dystocia, the impaction of the fetal anterior shoulder behind the maternal pubic symphysis, is an obstetric emergency that may be encountered in the ED during a precipitous delivery. How is the diagnosis made?

肩位难产是指胎儿前肩嵌顿在产妇耻骨联合后面，是可能在急诊科紧急分娩时遇到的产科急症。如何作出诊断？

The diagnosis is made if the clinician is unable to deliver the fetal anterior shoulder with downward traction on the fetal head or, after delivery of the head, the fetal chin retracts back onto the maternal perineum("turtle sign").

可通过如下方法作出诊断，如果医生不能通过将胎头向下牵引牵出胎儿的前肩或在胎儿头部牵出后，胎儿的下颌部缩回到产妇的阴道内（"乌龟征"），则可诊断为"肩位难产"（*J Emerg Med*, 2014, 46：378）。

301. 妊娠与下腔静脉

At what gestational age does the gravid uterus reach a size the will compromise aortocaval blood flow and cardiac output?

在妊娠的什么时期子宫的大小将影响主动脉和下腔静脉的血流量及心排血量？

At a gestation age of 20 weeks and beyond, the pregnant uterus can press against the IVC and aorta, impeding venous return.

在胎龄 20 周以后，妊娠子宫将压迫下腔静脉和主动脉，阻碍静脉回流 (*Circulation*, 2005, 112: 150)。

302. 葡萄胎妊娠

What is a hydatidiform mole (molar pregnancy)? How do they typically present?

什么是葡萄胎(葡萄胎妊娠)？通常的临床表现是什么？

A hydatidiform mole is a benign tumor of placental trophoblastic cells, which release human chorionic gonadotropin (hCG). The most common presentation is vaginal bleeding with high levels of hCG.

葡萄胎是一种良性的胎盘滋养层细胞肿瘤，释放人类绒毛膜促性腺激素 (HCG)。最常见的临床表现是妊娠后子宫大小与妊期不成比例，阴道出血和 HCG 水平升高 (*J Emerg Med*, 2014, 46: 348)。

303. 腹腔宫外孕的机制

What is the mechanism by which most abdominal ectopic pregnancies occur?

多数腹腔宫外孕的机制是什么？

Most abdominal pregnancies are secondary (i. e. result from the reimplantation of a ruptured tubal or ampullary pregnancy). A small proportion are primary, with normal Fallopian tubes and adnexa and no evidence of injury.

大多数腹腔妊娠是继发的(即由于一个破裂的输卵管壶腹部妊娠再植造成的)。只有一小部分是原发的,其输卵管及附件都正常,没有损伤的证据(*J Emerg Med*, 2006, 30: 171)。

 ## 304. 卵巢扭转与妊娠

Can ovarian torsion occur during pregnancy?

在怀孕期间可以发生卵巢扭转吗?

Up to 1/5 of ovarian torsion occurs during pregnancy. Ovarian torsion is most common in the 1st trimester; torsion early in pregnancy seems to increase the risk for recurrence at a later gestational age.

高达 1/5 的卵巢扭转发生在怀孕期间。卵巢扭转在第一孕期最常见,怀孕早期扭转将增加怀孕后期再出现扭转的风险(*J Emerg Med*, 2013, 46: 348)。

 ## 305. 子痫常发生在妊娠期的哪个阶段?

At what gestational age is eclampsia most often seen?

子痫最常发生在妊娠期的哪个阶段?

Rarely seen before 20 weeks gestation, eclampsia is most often seen in the late third trimester.

子痫很少在妊娠 20 周前发生,最常见于妊娠晚期的后期(*J Emerg Med*, 2008, 34: 199)。

306. 控制子痫惊厥的首选药物

Prompt delivery is considered to be the only definitive treatment for eclampsia. Before delivery, treatment consists of controlling seizure activity and lowering BP. What is the first drug administered? What is the dose?

立即分娩被认为是唯一彻底治疗子痫惊厥的方法。分娩前，要进行控制癫痫样发作和降低血压的治疗。首选药物是什么？多大剂量？

Magnesium sulfate is the first drug administered and is the mainstay for seizure control. The initial dose is 4 to 6 grams of magnesium sulfate IV, followed by a drip at a dose of 2 grams per hour.

硫酸镁是首选药物，是控制癫痫样发作的主要方法。初始剂量为静脉注射 4～6 g 硫酸镁，随后以每小时 2 g 的剂量静脉滴注(*J Emerg Med*, 2008, 34：199)。

 307. 产后子痫

Eclamptic convulsions can occur before, during, or after delivery. Postpartum eclampsia occurs in 10 – 45% of women with eclampsia. How long after delivery can eclamptic convulsions occur?

子痫抽搐可以在分娩前期、中期或后期发生。10%～45% 患有癫痫病怀孕的妇女会发生产后子痫。分娩后多久可以发生子痫抽搐？

About half of the cases of postpartum eclampsia occur within 48 hours after delivery, and the remainder occur between 2 days and 4 weeks after delivery (delayed postpartum eclampsia).

约有一半的产后子痫发生在产后 48 小时内，其余的在产后 2 天和 4 周(延迟产后子痫)之间出现 (*N Engl J Med*, 2009, 360：1126)。

308.带状疱疹的愈合时间

The lesions of herpes zoster go through stages, beginning as red macules and papules that, in the course of 7 – 10 days, evolve into vesicles and form pustules and crusts. How long does complete healing take?

带状疱疹的病变经历不同的阶段，开始为红色的斑疹和丘疹，在 7 ~ 10 天的过程中，演变成疱疹并形成小脓疱和结痂。完全愈合需要多久？

Complete healing may take more than 4 weeks.

带状疱疹完全愈合可能需要超过 4 周的时间（*Mayo Clin Proc*，2009，84：274）。

 309.带状疱疹的传染性

When in the course of the illness is shingles contagious? Is it more or less contagious that chickenpox?

在带状疱疹的发病过程中，什么时候具有传染性？与水痘相比，它的传染性是高还是低？

Less contagious than primary varicella, herpes zoster is only contagious after the rash appears and until the lesions crust. Risk of transmission is reduced further if lesions are covered

与原发性水痘相比，带状疱疹的传染性低，通常在皮疹出现后直至病变结痂。覆盖病变会使传播的危险性降低（*Mayo Clin Proc*，2009，84：274）。

310. 带状疱疹的易感人群

Persons with localized zoster should avoid contact with susceptible persons at high risk for severe varicella until lesions are crusted. What groups compromise such susceptible persons?

局部带状疱疹患者应避免与严重水痘易感者接触，直到病灶结痂。哪些人属于这样的易感者？

Such persons include pregnant women, all premature infants born to susceptible mothers, infants born at < 28 weeks' gestation or who weigh < 1000 gregardless of maternal immune status, and immunocompromised persons of all ages.

易感人群包括孕妇，所有易感母亲的早产儿。不论母亲免疫状态如何，28 周前出生的新生儿或低体重儿（体质量 <1 kg 的婴儿）和所有年龄段免疫功能低下者（*MMWR Weekly*，2008，57：1）。

311. 带状疱疹的抗病毒治疗

In controlled trials, antiviral therapy for herpes zoster has been initiated within 72 hours after rash onset. When should the clinician be prompted to start therapy even if the patient's rash began more than 3 days earlier?

在对照试验中，带状疱疹抗病毒治疗要在皮疹出现后 72 小时内开始。在什么情况下，即使患者的皮疹已超过 3 天，医生也应该及时开始治疗？

Many experts recommend that if new skin lesions are still appearing or complications of herpes zoster are present, treatment should be initiated even if the rash began more than 3 days earlier.

许多专家建议，如果仍然有新的皮疹出现或发生带状疱疹的并发症，即使皮疹超过 3 天也要开始抗病毒治疗（*N Engl J Med*，2013，369：255）。

312. 导致疥疮皮疹的原因

Scabies is caused by infestation of the epidermis with the mite Sarcoptes scabiei, variety hominis. What causes the rash of scabies?

疥疮是由各种人型螨（疥螨）侵入表皮引起的。导致疥疮皮疹（图43）的原因是什么？

The rash is due to hypersensitivity reaction to the mite protein.

皮疹是由对螨蛋白高度过敏反应引起的（*Mayo Clin Proc*, 2012, 87: 695）。

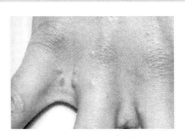

图43　导致指蹼间的疥疮皮疹

 313. 患疥疮后瘙痒会持续多久？

How long can pruritis last after treatment of scabies?

疥疮治疗后瘙痒会持续多久？

Pruritis can persist for up to 4 weeks after the end of correctly administered scabicide therapy. After that time, the cause of itching should be reinvestigated.

瘙痒可以在疥疮有效治疗结束后持续长达4周。超过这个时间，应该寻找造成瘙痒的其他原因（*N Engl J Med*, 2006, 354: 1718）。

314. 固定性药疹

What is a fixed drug eruption?

什么是固定性药疹?

A fixed drug eruption is an erythema multiforme-like adverse drug reaction that occurs in the same location each time the person uses a particular medication.

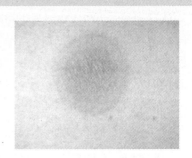

固定性药疹(图44)是当一个人在每次使用特定的药物后在同一个位置出现多形红斑样的药物不良反应。(*MMWR Weekly*, 2013, 62:914)

图44 固定性药疹

 315. DRESS 综合征

What syndrome is characterized by skin rash, fever, pharyngitis, lymphadenopathy, and visceral organ involvement presenting within 8 weeks of initiation of, typically, anti-convulsant therapy? What 2 anti-convulsants are usually the cause?

什么综合征通常在使用抗惊厥药8周内出现,其临床特征为皮疹、发热、咽喉炎、淋巴结肿大、内脏器官受累? 导致这种综合征常用的2种抗惊厥药是什么?

Drug rash with eosinophilia and systemic symptoms (DRESS) syndrome is estimated to occur in at least 1 per 1500 new users of phenytoin and carbamazepine.

药物皮疹,嗜酸性粒细胞增多和全身症状(DRESS)综合征是使用抗惊厥药最易出现的综合征,估计至少在 1/1500 的患者会发生此综合征。常在使用苯妥英钠和卡马西平的患者中发生(*J Emerg Med*, 2013, 44:75)。

316. A 组链球菌咽炎诊断试验（1）

Why are diagnostic studies for group A streptococcal pharyngitis are usually not indicated for children <3 years old?

为什么小于 3 岁儿童不必要做 A 组链球菌咽炎诊断试验？

Testing for GAS pharyngitis in children <3 years is usually not indicated since ARF is rare in such children and the incidence of streptococcal pharyngitis and its classic presentation are uncommon in this age group.

小于 3 岁儿童通常不必要做 A 组链球菌咽炎诊断试验，因为在这一年龄段，急性肾衰竭的发生率很低，并且链球菌咽炎的发病率及其典型表现是罕见的（*Clin Infect Dis*, 2012, 55: 1279）。

317. A 组链球菌咽炎诊断试验（2）

IDSA guidelines state that testing for GAS pharyngitis is usually not indicated for children <3 years old since the prevalence of GAS is low as is the risk of developing ARF. When might it be reasonable to test symptomatic children <3 years of age?

美国传染病学会不建议对小于 3 岁的儿童做链球菌咽炎检查，因为这一年龄的链球菌感染发生率和产生急性肾衰竭的危险性小。但什么时候需要对有症状的小于 3 岁儿童做检查？

If there is household contact with a school-aged sibling with documented strep pharyngitis, it is reasonable to test a symptomatic child. This is also true of a child in a day care with a high rate of GAS infections.

如果家里有一个患有链球菌咽炎的学龄期兄弟姐妹，应该对这个家庭内小于 3 岁的孩子做检查。同样，要对一个链球菌感染率高的幼儿园孩子做检查（*Clin Infect Dis*, 2012, 55: 1279）。

318. A 组链球菌咽炎(3)

When an antibiotic is prescribed for streptococcal pharyngitis, a clinical response is usually seen in 24 – 48 hours. Even without treatment, symptomscommonly resolve within a few days. What does the persistence of symptoms beyond this period suggest?

当用抗生素治疗链球菌咽炎时,临床效果通常在 24~48 小时出现。即使不治疗,症状也通常在几天内缓解。如果症状持续超过这个期限将提示什么?

Persistent symptoms beyond this period suggests either the development of a suppurative complication or that the patient may be a chronic carrier of GAS (not acutely infected)with an intercurrent viral pharyngitis.

如果症状持续超过这个时间说明发生了化脓性并发症,或患者是慢性携带者(非急性感染)合并有病毒性咽炎(*Clin Infect Dis*, 2012, 55: 1279)。

319. 对青霉素过敏患者咽炎的治疗

What is appropriate treatment of group A streptococcal pharyngitis in penicillin-allergic individuals?

治疗对青霉素(PCN)过敏的链球菌(GAS)咽炎患者应该使用什么抗生素?

Treatment of GAS pharyngitis in PCN-allergic patients: A first generation cephalosporin (for those not anaphylactically sensitive) for 10 days, clindamycin or clarithromycin for 10 days, or azithromycin for 5 days.

治疗对青霉素(PCN)过敏的链球菌(GAS)咽炎患者:第一代头孢菌素治疗(对于那些没有过敏性休克的)10 天,克林霉素或克拉霉素治疗 10 天,或阿奇霉素治疗 5 天(*Clin Infect Dis*, 2012, 55: 1279)。

320. 急性中耳炎与 β – 内酰胺酶类抗生素

Amoxicillin is the first-line treatment for pediatric acute otitis media when a decision to treat with antibiotics is made; however, when should clinicians prescribe an antibiotic with additional Beta-lactamase coverage?

在决定用抗生素治疗小儿急性中耳炎后，阿莫西林是第一线的抗生素。但是，在什么情况下医生需要用 β – 内酰胺酶类抗生素？

Prescribe an antibiotic with additional Beta-lactamase coverage if the child has received amoxicillin in the last 30 days, has concurrent purulent conjunctivitis, orhas a history of recurrent AOM unresponsive to amoxicillin.

如果孩子已经在过去 30 天内用过阿莫西林，或合并有化脓性结膜炎，或有对阿莫西林无反应而复发的急性中耳炎的病史，要用 β – 内酰胺酶类抗生素（*Pediatrics*, 2013, 131：e964）。

321. 急性中耳炎做鼓膜置管术的指征

Emergency physicians often see children with repeat visits for acute otitis media, and parents may inquire about the role of tympanostomy. When is tympanostomyinidcated?

急诊医师经常看到儿童因急性中耳炎（AOM）复发就诊，家长可能会咨询鼓膜置管术的作用。什么时候应考虑做鼓膜置管术？

Clinicians may offer tympanostomy tubes for recurrent AOM (3 episodes in 6 months or 4 episodes in 1 year with 1 episode in the preceding 6 months).

对于复发性急性中耳炎（6 个月复发 3 次，或 1 年内复发 4 次，其中 6 个月内有 1 次复发），临床医生可能会建议做鼓膜置管术（*Pediatrics*, 2013, 131：e964）。

322. 严重急性细菌性鼻窦炎

According to IDSA guidelines, "high-dose" (2 g orally bid or 90 mg/kg/day orally bid) amoxicillin-clavulanate is recommended for acute bacterial rhinosinusitis for those with severe infection. What defines a severe infection?

根据美国传染病学会(IDSA)指南：大剂量阿莫西林 - 克拉维酸(每天每公斤体重 90 mg，每日分 2 次口服；或 2000 mg，每日分 2 次口服)可用于治疗严重急性细菌性鼻窦炎感染。严重的感染是如何定义的?

Systemic toxicity with fever of at least102℉ and threat of suppurative complications, daycare attendance, age ＜ 2 or ＞ 65 years, recent hospitalization, antibiotic use within the past month, or immunocompromised state.

具有下列全身毒性表现：体温至少 102℉(38.9℃)，有化脓性并发症，是上托儿所的儿童，年龄 <2 岁或 >65 岁，最近住过院，在过去的一个月内用过抗生素，或免疫功能低下(*Clin Infect Dis*，2012，54：e72)。

323. 单眼漂浮物感和(或)闪光感

What is the cause of most cases of acute-onset monocular floaters and/or flashes?

急性发作的单眼漂浮物感和(或)闪光感的最常见的原因是什么?

Posterior vitreous detachment.

后部玻璃体脱离(*JAMA*，2009，302：2243)。

324. 急性视网膜剥脱的典型临床表现

What is the classic description of the presenting symptoms by a patient experiencing an acute retinal detachment?

急性视网膜剥脱患者的典型临床表现是什么?

Classically, patients describe a sudden, painless, monocular visual impairment with the sensation of looking through a curtain, accompanied by flashes and floaters.

急性视网膜剥脱的患者典型的主诉为突发的,无痛性的,单侧视力改变,像通过门帘视物,有闪光和漂浮物的感觉(*Ann Emerg Med*, 2015, In Press)。

 ## 325. 视神经炎的临床表现

What are the presenting signs and symptoms of optic neuritis?

视神经炎的症状和体征是什么?

Presenting signs and symptoms include decreased visual acuity in the affected eye, ocular pain that is exacerbated by eye movements and a relative afferent pupillary defect on examination.

视神经炎的症状和体征包括患侧眼视力下降,眼痛并随眼球活动加重,并在体检时有相对性瞳孔传入反射异常(马库斯·冈恩瞳孔,Marcus Gunn pupil)(*J Emerg Med*, 2014, 47: 301)。

 ## 326. 急性青光眼的典型临床表现

What are the typical clinical findings associated with acute glaucoma?

什么是急性青光眼的典型临床表现?

On exam, there will be decreased visual acuity, a mid-dilated sluggishly reactive or non-reactive pupil, a red-injected conjunctiva, and a shallow anterior chamber. The hallmark is an intraocular pressure >21 mm Hg.

体检时会有视力下降、管视、瞳孔中度缩小并对光反应迟钝或无反应,结膜发红充血和眼前房变窄。最主要的标志是眼压 >21 mmHg(*J Emerg Med*, 2013, 44: 1143)。

327. 一过性黑矇

Exactly what is amaurosis fugax?

一过性黑矇(amaurosis fugax)究竟是什么?

Emboli in retinal arterioles lead to transient monocular blindness (amaurosisfugax) The most common source of these emboli is an atherosclerotic carotid artery.

视网膜小动脉栓塞导致短暂的单眼失明(一过性黑矇)。这些栓子最常来源是颈动脉粥样硬化(*N Engl J Med*, 2013, 369: 1718)。

328. 流行性角结膜炎

Epidemic keratoconjunctivitis is a highly contagious, severe form of conjunctivitis, often caused by adenovirus. Symptoms include a gritty feeling in the eyes, watery discharge, photophobia, and redness. For how long do symptoms typically last?

流行性角结膜炎是一种具有高度传染性,由腺病毒引起的严重结膜炎的一种眼病。症状包括眼里有沙粒样感觉、水样分泌物、畏光和红肿。症状通常会持续多久?

Clinical illness typically lasts 7 – 21 days and is usually self-limited. Corneal involvement, including keratitis and subepithelial infiltrates, can persist for months, affecting visual acuity.

临床表现通常持续7~21天,一般是自限性的。角膜受累,包括角膜炎和表皮下浸润,可以持续数月,最终影响视力(*MMWR Weekly*, 2013, 62: 637)。

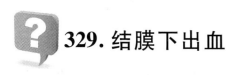

329. 结膜下出血

Subconjunctival hemorrhage is not uncommonly seen in patients presenting to the ED. A high-profile hemorrhage will take 10 – 14 days to resolve. What treatments can be recommended to reduce the recovery time?

因结膜下出血（图45）到急诊科就诊的患者并不是不常见的。严重的出血将需要10～14天才能消失。建议用什么治疗方法可以缩短恢复时间？

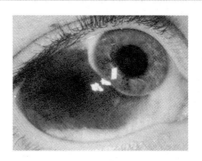

图45　结膜下出血

Prescribing warm compresses and lubrication drops will help reduce recovery by 1 – 3 days.

热敷和润滑眼药水会将恢复时间缩短1～3天（*EMCNA*，2013，26：35）。

330. 乙酰氨基酚中毒导致急性肝功能衰竭的危险

What two groups of patients are at increased risk of acute liver failure due to acetaminophen-induced hepatotoxicity?

哪两种患者在乙酰氨基酚中毒引起肝损害时导致急性肝功能衰竭的危险性高？

Malnourished patients and patients with alcoholism are at increased risk.

营养不良和酗酒患者的危险性增高（*N Engl J Med*，2013，369：2526）。

 ## 331. 乙酰氨基酚中毒的死亡率

Is death from an acetaminophen ingestion more likely to occur after a single large dose or a staggered ingestion over hours or days?

一次服用大剂量乙酰氨基酚中毒的死亡率要比几小时或几天内分次服用的死亡率高吗？

Although acute liver failure after APAP ingestion can occur after ingestion of a single large dose, the risk of death is greatest with substantial drug ingestion staggered over hours or days rather than at a single time point.

虽然在一次大剂量服用乙酰氨基酚后可出现急性肝衰竭，但死亡的风险在几小时或几天内分次大量服用是最高的，而不是单一时间点的一次性服用（*N Engl J Med*，2013，369：2526）。

332. 急性水杨酸中毒

What is the significance of clinical deterioration due to acute salicylate toxicitiy in the setting of a falling serum concentration?

在急性水杨酸中毒时，血清浓度下降但临床症状却恶化的意义是什么？

Deterioration, even with a falling serum concentration, is ominous and suggests increasing CNS salicylate concentration. As blood pH falls, there is more nonionized salicylate to readily distribute into the CSF.

血清水杨酸浓度下降但临床症状却出现恶化，是一个不良征兆，提示中枢神经系统内水杨酸浓度的增加。在血液的 pH 下降时，更多的非游离水杨酸渗透到脑脊液中（*Am Coll Med Toxicol Guideline*, 2013）。

333. 如何碱化水杨酸中毒患者的尿液？

Urine alkalinization to a pH of 7.5 – 8.0 increases salicylate excretion > 10 – fold and should be considered for significant salicylate toxicity in patients with intact renal function. How is urinary alkalinization achieved in such cases?

将尿液碱化到 pH 为 7.5 ~ 8.0 可使水杨酸排泄率增加 10 倍以上，所以，碱化尿液应该用于肾功能正常的水杨酸中毒患者。在这种情况下，如何达到尿液碱化的目的？

One commonly utilized IV solution consists of 1 liter of D5W to which 3 50 mL – ampules of 8.4% sodium bicarbonate and 30 – 40 mEq of KCl/L are added. The rate of infusion should be sufficient to induce a urine output of 2 – 3 mL/kg/hr.

一种普遍用于尿液碱化的液体是将 8.4% 碳酸氢钠注射液 150 mL 和 30 ~ 40 mEg 氯化钾注射液加入 1000 mL 的 5% 葡萄糖注射液中所得到的混合溶液，然后静脉滴注。输液的速度应该使尿量达到 2 ~ 3 mL/（kg · h）（*Am Coll Med Toxicol Guideline*, 2013）。

334."浴盐"的名字是如何来的？

How did the name "bath salts" originate?

"浴盐"的名字是如何起源的？

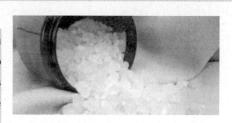

The name originated in the UK when the drugs became illegal there. In order to avoid the law, dealers marketed the drugs using the name bath salts as the crystalline drugs resemble sodium chloride bath salts.

图46　"浴盐"

"浴盐"这个名字起源于英国，当时认为此盐是毒品，在英国是非法的。为了避免法律限制，药贩子将此毒品以"浴盐"的名字进入市场，因为此药的晶体状类似于洗浴用的氯化钠，见图46(*N Engl J Med*, 2013, 369: 2545)。

 335."浴盐"是由什么化学物衍生的？

"Bath Salts" are synthetic derivatives of what chemical?

"浴盐"是由什么化学物衍生的？

"Bath Salts" are synthetic derivatives of cathinone, a sympathomimetic chemical found in the leaves of the khat plant (Catha edulis). The use of bath salts is associated with sympathomimetic activity and psychotic behavior.

"浴盐"是卡西酮的合成衍生物，卡西酮是在卡塔叶植物(Catha 牛肝菌)的叶子中发现的一种使交感神经兴奋的化学物质。使用"浴盐"可产生与拟交感神经亢进和精神病类似的行为(*N Engl J Med*, 2013, 369: 2545)。

336. "浴盐"作用的持续时间

The toxic effects of "bath salts" are largely the same as those seen in patients who have taken large doses of amphetamines. For how long do the effects last?

"浴盐"的毒性作用在绝大部分上与服用大量安非他明的患者相同。其作用会持续多久？

The primary psychological effects have a duration of roughly 3 – 4 hrs, with physiologic effects such as tachycardia, hypertension, and mild stimulation lasting 6 – 8 hrs.

主要的精神情绪影响会持续大约 3 ~ 4 小时，而生理效应，如心动过速、高血压、轻度兴奋可持续 6 ~ 8 小时（*J Emerg Med*, 2013, 45: 364）。

讨论："浴盐"

概况	近两年出现的新型"designer drug"（合成毒品）毒品。
性状	这种毒品并不是真正放到浴缸里用的盐，只是白色的、晶体状、类似于盐的一种毒品。
成分	一个研究发现，在 130 个样品中，有 254 种不同的化学成分，48 个不同的组合。主要成分包括 cathinones methylenedioxypyrovalerone（MDPV），4 – methylmethcathinone（methylone，4 – MMC），3, 4 – methylenedioxymethcathinone（mephedrone）和咖啡因，利多卡因，冰毒，吗啡等。
用法	可鼻吸，食入或静脉注射。

337. 食入过氧化氢的危险

Hydrogen peroxide is sold in health-food stores in a 35% solution as a cleansing agent for "hyperoxygenation" therapy. Why can ingestion of this agent result in neurologic syndromes (mimicking stroke deficits, from paresthesias to obtundation)?

在健康食品商店出售的 35% 过氧化氢溶液被作为"高氧化"清洁剂使用。为什么食入这种试剂会导致神经系统症状（类似于脑卒中的表现，从感觉异常到反应迟钝)?

With 35% H₂O₂, each mL produces 100 mL of O₂ gas. Such gas formation can be life threatening, producing cerebral and portal venous emboli. There are multiple case reports of successful treatment with hyperbaric oxygen therapy.

每毫升的 35% 过氧化氢可产生 100 mL 氧气。这种气体的产生可危及生命，造成脑和门静脉栓子。已有多例用高压氧治疗成功的报告(*J Emerg Med*, 2014, 46: 171)。

 338. 过氧化氢摄入导致的气体栓塞

Hydrogen peroxide ingestion can result in gas embolization, from either direct dissection of oxygen from the GI tract into tissues or from conversion of hydrogen peroxide absorbed into the circulatory system. What treatment is available?

过氧化氢的摄入可以导致气体栓塞，可能是由于氧直接从胃肠道进入组织或吸收后进入循环系统的过氧化氢的转换引起。目前有哪些治疗方法？

Hyperbaric oxygen (HBO) therapy, traditionally used for the treatment of gas emboli caused by rapid ascent while diving, has also been used to treat emboli produced by hydrogen peroxide ingestion.

传统上用于治疗潜水时快速上升所造成气体栓塞的高压氧(HBO)治疗，也可以用来治疗过氧化氢摄入所产生的气体栓塞(*J Emerg Med*, 2013, 45: 346)。

 339. 一氧化碳中毒的高压氧治疗

In a recent study of patients with intentional CO poisoning, almost half had a co-ingestion-most commonly ethanol. Why is it so important to keep this in mind in the ED?

在最近的一个有关故意一氧化碳(CO)中毒患者的研究中，几乎有一半患者同时摄入了其他相关品，最常见的是乙醇。为什么在急诊科记住这一点如此重要？

Indications for hyperbaric oxygen treatment include alteration of mental status; intoxication with ethanol can confuse the clinical picture and make the decision regarding hyperbaric oxygen treatment difficult.

高压氧治疗的适应证包括神志改变。乙醇中毒将混淆临床表现，对决定是否使用高压氧治疗增加了难度(*J Emerg Med*, 2013, 44: 625)。

340. 氰化物中毒的拮抗药

The traditional treatment for cyanide poisoning is a 3 - part kit of amyl nitrite, sodium nitrite, and sodium thiosulfate. The kits are not without drawbacks, and many experts recommend hydroxocobalamin as first-line therapy. What are the drawbacks?

传统的治疗氰化物中毒是亚硝酸戊酯、亚硝酸钠和硫代硫酸钠的三元急救盒。该急救盒治疗方法并不是没有缺点的，许多专家建议用羟钴胺作为一线治疗。此三元急救盒有哪些缺点？

Nitrite administration may cause hypotension and induction of MetHb may worsen the functional anemia present in patients with concurrent CO poisoning. The kit is complicated to administer and requires rapid dosage calculations.

亚硝酸盐的使用可能会导致低血压和继而产生的甲基血红蛋白，可能会使由合并一氧化碳中毒引起的功能性贫血加重。该急救盒的使用很复杂并需要快速计算剂量(*Am J Emerg Med*, 2012, 30: 231)。

341. 海洛因和奥施康定

The price paid for diverted pharmaceutical drugs is often considerably higher than an equipotent dose of heroin. A $10 packet of heroin compares pharmacodynamically with what dose of OxyContin?

不同商品药(鸦片制剂)的价格往往要比等效剂量的海洛因高出很多。一包10美元的海洛因相当于多大剂量的奥施康定？

Public health officials say that a ＄10 packet of heroin compares pharmacodynamically with a single 80 mg OxyContin pill worth approximately ＄80 on the street.

公共卫生官员透露，一包10美元的海洛因在药效动力学上相当于黑市上价值80美元的80 mg奥施康定(*Mayo Clin Proc*, 2014, 89: 437)。

 ## 342. 纳洛酮作用的持续时间

What is the duration of action of naloxone?

纳洛酮作用的持续时间是多长？

The duration of action of naloxone is approximately 45 to 70 minutes, but respiratory depression caused by ingestion of a long-acting opioid (eg, methadone) may last longer.

纳洛酮作用持续时间约45~70分钟，但由摄入一种长效阿片类药物(如美沙酮)所引起的呼吸抑制可能会持续更长的时间(*Circulation*, 2010, 122: S829)。

 ## 343. 这样吃鲭鱼安全吗？

Scombroid poisoning is caused by a bacterial overgrowth on fish that, at some point in the transit from the sea to the consumer, are not stored at an appropriately low temperature. Does cooking of the fish prevent scombroid poisoning?

鲭鱼中毒是由细菌过度污染的鱼所致，是由于在从海上到消费者过程中的某个环节没有适当的低温储存。烹调可以防止鲭鱼中毒吗？

Scombroid poisoning is a result of bacteria on the fish surface that decarboxylate histidine to histamine and other toxins, causing classical histaminergic symptoms. These toxins are not broken down by cooking.

鲭鱼中毒是由鱼表面感染了可将组氨酸脱羧成组胺和其他毒素的细菌所致，导致典型的组胺类症状。这些毒素不会因烹饪而破坏。(*J Emerg Med*, 2013, 45: 909)

讨论：鲭鱼中毒

1. 经常由食用冷藏不当的鲭鱼、金枪鱼、竹荚鱼、鲯鳅鱼、鲣鱼、沙丁鱼、凤尾鱼引起。

2. 新鲜的鱼不含有组胺,因此这些鱼在打捞后一定要速冻。如储存在0℃时,安全期为14天;4℃时为7天;4℃以上时不要超过4小时。

3. 症状和治疗与普通过敏反应一样。

4. 可通过组胺鉴定判断污染的鱼。

 344. 鲭鱼中毒

Symptoms of scombroid poisoning include urticarial, flushing, edema, paresthesia of the mouth, and abdominal pain. What is the underlying pathophysiology?

鲭鱼中毒的症状包括荨麻疹、潮红、浮肿、口周感觉异常和腹痛。其病理生理机制是什么?

Scombroid poisoning is caused by the consumption of inadequately preserved or refrigerated fish. Bacteria in the fish contain a decarboxylase enzyme that converts histidine to histamine, which is resistant to cooking and freezing.

鲭鱼中毒是因吃了保存或冷藏不当的鱼。在鱼里的细菌含有脱羧酶,将组氨酸转化为组胺,使细菌既耐蒸煮又抗冷冻(*N Engl J Med*, 2013, 368: e31)。

 345. 雪卡毒鱼中毒

Ciguatera fish poisoning is characterized by GI, cardiovascular, and neurologic symptoms and results from ingesting toxins that accumulate in coral reef fish (e. g., barracuda, grouper, snapper). When is symptom onset after eating contaminated fish?

雪卡毒鱼中毒(CFP)的特点是由摄入积聚在珊瑚礁鱼(例如梭鱼、石斑鱼、鲷鱼)的毒素引起的胃肠道、心血管和神经系统症状。这些症状通常在进食受污染的鱼多长时间后发作?

The majority of patients experience symptoms within 6 – 48 hours after eating contaminated fish. Initial treatment options for CFP are limited and supportive only.

多数患者吃污染的鱼后 6~48 小时内出现症状。雪卡毒鱼中毒(CFP)初始治疗选择是有限的，只有支持措施(*MMWR Weekly*, 2013, 62: 61)。

346. 甲醇中毒

Methanol is a relatively common and potentially fatal toxic alcohol ingestion. In what substances is methanol is commonly found?

甲醇中毒是摄入一种比较常见的和具有潜在致命毒性的酒精。甲醇通常发现于哪些物质里？

Methanol is commonly found in solvents, de-icers, glass cleaners, as well as homemade alcohols ("moonshine").

甲醇经常发现在溶剂、除冰剂、玻璃清洗剂以及自制的酒精("高度白酒")中(*Emerg Med Intern*, 2013, 2013: Article ID 638057)。

讨论：甲醇中毒

主要特点	视力改变，神经系统症状，代谢性酸中毒
主要治疗	碳酸氢钠，乙醇，fomepizole（甲吡唑）
血透指征	①摄入 30 mL 以上的甲醇；②血清甲醇水平超过 20 mg/dL；③视力丧失；④对碳酸氢钠无反应的代谢性酸中毒

347. 重症酒精戒断综合征

Initial treatment of severe alcohol withdrawal syndrome in the ED begins with IV loading of benzodiazepines. Loading doses of 1–4 mg of lorazepam should be given how often?

急诊重症酒精戒断综合征的治疗开始通常使用负荷量的静脉苯二氮卓类药物。1~4 mg 的劳拉西泮负荷剂量可以多长时间给一次？

Every 10–15 minutes. The appropriately treated patient has near-normal/normal vital signs and is calm, sleepy but arousable, no evidence of active hallucinations, and not seizing.

劳拉西泮每 10 ~ 15 分钟给予一次。治疗有效的患者应有接近正常或正常的生命体征并安静, 困倦, 但易唤醒, 没有任何幻觉的迹象, 同时又不发生抽搐(*Am J Emerg Med*, 2013, 31 : 734)。

348. 胰高血糖素治疗 β 受体阻滞药中毒的应用剂量

Administration of glucagon may be helpful for severe cardiovascular instability associated with Beta-blocker toxicity that is refractory to standard measures, including vasopressors. What is the recommended dose?

在治疗由 β 受体阻滞药中毒导致的严重的心血管功能不稳定; 但对常规措施(包括升压药)无反应时, 应用胰高血糖素可能会有帮助。它的推荐剂量是多少?

The recommended dose of glucagon is a bolus of 3 to 10 mg, administered slowly over 3 to 5 minutes, followed by an infusion of 3 to 5 mg/h (0. 05 to 0. 15 mg/kg followed by an infusion of 0. 05 to 0. 10 mg/kg/hr).

胰高血糖素的推荐剂量为 3 ~ 10 mg, 在 3 ~ 5 分钟内缓慢静脉注射, 随后以每小时 3 ~ 5 mg 的剂量静脉滴注(按每千克体重 0. 05 ~ 0. 15 mg 静脉注射, 然后以每小时每千克体重 0. 05 ~ 0. 10 mg 静脉滴注)(*Circulation*, 2010, 122 : S829)。

349. 高剂量胰岛素和静脉脂肪乳剂治疗 β 受体阻滞药和钙拮抗药中毒

Treatment of Beta-blocker and calcium-channel blocker overdose involves epinephrine, atropine, glucagon, and calcium, but these therapies are often ineffective in severe overdoses. What 2 treatment options have emerged for severe CCB and BB overdoses?

β受体阻滞药和钙拮抗药中毒的治疗包括肾上腺素、阿托品、胰高血糖素和钙制剂，但这些治疗对重症中毒通常是无效的。最近出现的两种用于β受体阻滞药和钙拮抗药中毒的治疗方案是什么？

High-dose insulin and intravenous lipid emulsion.

高剂量胰岛素和静脉脂肪乳剂（*J Emerg Med*, 2014, 46: 486）。

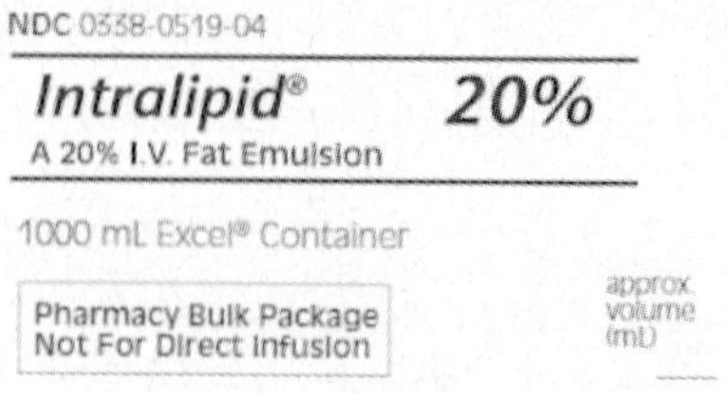

图 47 脂肪乳剂

讨论：使用方法

高剂量胰岛素	每公斤体重 1 单位静脉注射 然后每公斤体重每小时 1 单位静脉持续滴注
脂肪乳	20% 脂肪乳剂 1.5 mL/kg，静脉注射，然后以 0.25 mL/（kg·min）的滴速静脉滴注。

350. 地高辛抗体片段

Antidigoxin Fab antibodies should be administered to patients with life-threatening cardiac glycoside toxicity. In critical cases in which therapy is required before a serum digoxin level can be obtained, how many vials should be given empirically?

地高辛抗体片段应用于具有生命危险的强心苷中毒患者。在危急的情况下，需要在血清地高辛检测数据报告前就要给予地高辛抗体片段，应该给多少瓶的量？

In critical cases in which therapy is required before a serum digoxin level can be obtained or in cases of life-threatening toxicity due to cardiac glycosides, administer empirically 10 to 20 vials.

在危急或有生命危险的强心苷中毒情况下，需要在血清地高辛检测数据报告前就要给地高辛抗体片段，常规给予 10～20 瓶的量（*Circulation*, 2010, 122: S829）。

讨论：地高辛抗体片段

1 瓶地高辛抗体片段(又称 digibind)的用量可中和 0.5 mg 地高辛。

如已知患者的血清地高辛浓度为 3.0，那么患者将需要给予 4~5 瓶地高辛抗体片段的量。

另外一定要注意 K 和 Mg 的血清水平。

351. 这是什么中毒？

Symptoms of what poisoning include altered mental status and visual impairment with hyperemia and edema of the optic disc and may include infarction or hemorrhage of the basal ganglia?

什么中毒会有下列症状：神志改变，视神经盘充血和水肿造成的视力损伤，并还有可能产生包括基底节部位的梗死或出血？

Methanol Poisoning.

甲醇中毒(*Am J Emerg Med*, 2012, 30: 231)。

第十九篇　药物与治疗篇

 352. 青霉素过敏时可以用哪些头孢类抗生素？

Patients who are selectively allergic to amoxicillin should avoid cephalosporins that have similar R1-group side chains. Which cephalosporins should such patients avoid?

对阿莫西林选择性过敏的患者应避免使用有类似 R1 组侧链的头孢菌素。这些患者应避免哪些此类的头孢菌素？

Cephalexin, Cefaclor, Cefadroxil, Cefprozil, Cephradine, and Cefatrizine.

头孢氨苄，头孢克洛，头孢羟氨苄，头孢丙烯，头孢拉定和头孢硫脒（*J Emerg Med*, 2012, 42：612）。

 353. 氯胺酮升高眼内压的原因

Ketamine, a widely used agent for ED pediatric procedural sedation, is sympathomimetic and often increases pulse rate and blood pressure. It can also elevate intraocular pressure. By what mechanism does this occur?

氯胺酮，一种在急诊科广泛使用的儿科镇静的药物，具有拟交感神经作用，通常会增加脉率和血压。同时它还可以提高眼内压，这种作用是通过何种机制产生的？

Ketamine elevates IOP either as a result of general blood pressure elevation or tension in the extraocular muscles.

氯胺酮升高眼内压是血压或眼外肌张力增加的结果（*Ann Emerg Med*, 2014, 64：385）。

354. 丙泊酚和绿色尿

What parenteral drug commonly used in Emergency Medicine practice is known to turn the color of urine green?

急诊医学实践中常用的哪些肠外药物可以使尿变绿色?

Propofol. Although reported most frequently after prolonged infusions, it can happen following a single dose. Alkalinization of the urine favors the formation of the metabolites responsible for the green discoloration.

丙泊酚,虽然报道最多的是在长时间静脉用药后,但也可能发生在一次性使用之后。碱化尿液将有助于产生使尿变绿色的代谢产物(*Anesthesiol*,2012,116:924)。

355. 美国最常用的处方药

What is the most commonly prescribed medication in the US?

什么是美国最常用的处方药?

Hydrocodone is now the most commonly prescribed medication in the US, more than any blood pressure, cholesterol, or diabetes medication.

氢可酮(Hydrocodone)是目前在美国最常用的处方药,超过任何降血压、降胆固醇或治疗糖尿病的药物(*Am J Emerg Med*,2014,32:580)。

356. 冷冻血浆纠正华法林抗凝效应的剂量

What is the dose of FFP for reversal of warfarin anticoagulation?

冷冻血浆(FFP)纠正华法林抗凝效应的剂量是什么?

Although the optimal dose has not been established, FFP is most often administered in a dose of 15 mL/kg.

尽管冷冻血浆（FFP）的最佳剂量尚未确定，但 FFP 最经常应用的剂量是 15 mL/kg（*Am J Hematol*，2008，83：137）。

 ## 357. 冷冻血浆治疗 ACEI 所致血管性水肿的机制

What is the rationale for the use of FFP for the treatment of ACEI-induced angioedema?

使用冷冻血浆（FFP）治疗 ACEI 诱发的血管性水肿的基本原理是什么？

The proposed mechanism of ACEI-induced angioedema is the accumulation of bradykinin in plasma and tissues. FFP contains kininase II which is identical to ACE and catalyzes the degradation of excessive bradykinin.

ACEI 诱发的血管性水肿被认为可能是由缓激肽在血浆和组织中的积累所致。冷冻血浆含有与血管紧张素转换酶（ACE）相同的激肽酶 II，它可催化降解过多的缓激肽（*J Emerg Med*，2013，44：764）。

 ## 358. 肝素与血钾

Whether administered subcutaneously or intravenously, heparin has been shown to cause what electrolyte abnormality?

不论皮下或静脉内给药，已证明肝素可造成什么样的电解质紊乱？

Heparin decreases plasma aldosterone concentrations, leading to increases in measured serum potassium levels.

肝素可降低血浆醛固酮浓度，从而增加血钾水平（*Mayo Clin Proc*，2010，85：1046）。

359. 磺胺和钾及肌酐

What commonly prescribed antibiotic causes reversible elevation of serum potassium and creatinine levels?

哪种常用的处方抗生素可造成可逆性的血钾和肌酐水平升高?

The trimethoprim component of trimethoprim-sulfamethoxazole.

复方新诺明(磺胺)组成部分中的甲氧苄啶(*Mayo Clin Proc*, 2011, 86: 70)。

360. 哪些药物可出现光敏感反应?

Photosensitivity from systemic medications are almost always a consequence of UV or visible-light activation of a drug, resulting in a sunburn-like reaction that may blister in exposed areas. What drugs are commonly associated with phototoxicity?

由全身用药产生的光敏感反应几乎都是由一种药物通过紫外线或可见光激活后的结果,导致阳光晒黑样的反应,可在曝光部位形成水泡。光毒性通常与哪些药物有关?

Drugs commonly associated with phototoxicity include tetracyclines (particularly doxycycline), thiazide diuretics, quinolones, voriconazole, amiodarone, and vemurafenib.

通常产生光敏感反应的药物包括四环素类(特别是强力霉素)、噻嗪类利尿药、喹诺酮类、伏立康唑、胺碘酮、威罗菲尼 (*N Engl J Med*, 2012, 366: 2492)。

361. 急性高原病

What is the cardinal symptom of acute mountain sickness?

急性高原病的主要症状是什么?

Headache that occurs with an increase in altitude is the cardinal symptom of acute mountain sickness and is usually accompanied by anorexia, nausea, dizziness, malaise, sleep disturbance, or a combination of these symptoms.

随海拔高度的增加出现头痛是急性高原病的主要症状,通常伴有厌食、恶心、头晕、乏力、睡眠障碍,或这些症状的组合(*N Engl J Med*, 2013, 368:2294)。

362. "生理盐水"名称的来由

Emergency Physicians routinely use Normal Saline as the resuscitation intravenous fluid of choice. Why is it called "normal"?

急诊医师经常使用生理盐水作为首选的静脉复苏液体。为什么把这种盐水称为"生理(正常)"?

Saline's designation as "normal" was based on an erroneous calculation of the salt concentration in human blood as 0.9% back in 1882 (it's actually 0.6%).

之所以把这种盐水称为"生理(正常)",是由于在 1882 年对人血液盐浓度进行计算时错误地计算成了 0.9%,它实际上的盐浓度是 0.6%(*N Engl J Med*, 2013, 369: 1243)。

363. 髂肋综合征

Patients with osteoporosis may develop abdominal pain due to the iliocostal syndrome. What is the underlying mechanism of the pain?

骨质疏松症患者可出现腹部疼痛,称为髂肋综合征。疼痛的基本机制是什么?

With osteoporosis, vertebral compression fractures often result in a narrowing of the distance between the lowest anterior rib (the 10th rib) and the top of the iliac crest producing pain where this rib contacts the pelvis.

患有骨质疏松症患者,椎体压缩性骨折往往导致最低的前肋(第 10 肋骨)和髂嵴的距离变窄,当肋骨触及骨盆时可产生疼痛(*Mayo Clin Proc*, 2013, 88: 106)。

364. 抽血检查造成的血液丢失

Is blood loss due to diagnostic phlebotomy an important cause of anemia in hospitalized patients?

由于诊断性血液检测造成的血液丢失是住院患者贫血的一个重要原因吗?

Normal adult RBC production is 0.25 mL/kg/day, which is about 0.5 L of blood/week. Phlebotomy results in mean daily loss of up to 70 mL of blood in an ICU patient, which may be more than can be replaced in an ICU patient.

正常成人每天红细胞产生量为 0.25 mL/kg,相当于每周约 0.5 升血。如果一位危重症监护病室(ICU)的患者因诊断性血液检查造成的血液丢失平均每天高达 70 mL,这很可能高于其患者的代偿量(*Am J Crit Care*,2013,22:eS1)。

讨论:减少患者每天抽血量的方法

1. 应用儿科采血样试管

2. 减少动脉导管血液丢失

3. 减少不必要的血气分析(利用末梢氧饱和度监测和 $ETCO_2$)

4. 无创性血红蛋白监测

 365. 什么是假性动脉瘤?

Exactly what is a pseudoaneurysm?

什么是假性动脉瘤?

A pseudoaneurysm is created by arterial wall disruption leading to blood dissecting into surrounding tissues, resulting in a hematoma that communicates with the arterial lumen.

假性动脉瘤是由于动脉壁破裂后血液进入周围组织而导致的并与动脉管腔连通的血肿(*J Emerg Med*,2013,45:e171)。

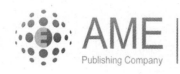

AME | Academic Made Easy, Excellent and Enthusiastic
Publishing Company | 砺窘千里目，快乐搞学术